BRCA1 and BRCA2 Mutations - Diagnostic and Therapeutic Implications

Edited by Mani T. Valarmathi

Published in London, United Kingdom

BRCA1 and BRCA2 Mutations - Diagnostic and Therapeutic Implications
http://dx.doi.org/10.5772/intechopen.100842
Edited by Mani T. Valarmathi

Contributors
Mani T. Valarmathi, Divya Bhargavi Pulukuri, Shanker Kalakotla, Vijaya Babu Penke, Divya Jyothi Palati, Prudvi Raj Pulla, Siddhartha Lolla, Sonali Verma, Gresh Chander, Ruchi Shah, Rakesh Kumar, Gvantsa Kharaishvili, Mariam Kacheishvili, Giorgi Akhvlediani, Rosa Maria Alvarez Gomez, Yuliana Sanchez Contreras, Brigney Isvettia Aceves Poveda, David Neri Acosta Gutierrez, Yousef M. Hawsawi, Anwar Shams, Edith C. Kordon, Natalia B. Burachik, Ana Laura Ortiz, Carlos Arturo Gonzalez Nuñez, Paula Anel Cabrera Galeana, Sandy Ruiz Cruz, Alexandra Garcilazo Reyes

First published in London, United Kingdom, 2023 by IntechOpen
IntechOpen is the global imprint of INTECHOPEN LIMITED, registered in England and Wales, registration number: 11086078, 5 Princes Gate Court, London, SW7 2QJ, United Kingdom

British Library Cataloguing-in-Publication Data
A catalogue record for this book is available from the British Library

Additional hard and PDF copies can be obtained from orders@intechopen.com

BRCA1 and BRCA2 Mutations - Diagnostic and Therapeutic Implications
Edited by Mani T. Valarmathi
p. cm.
Print ISBN 978-1-80356-806-5
Online ISBN 978-1-80356-807-2
eBook (PDF) ISBN 978-1-80356-808-9

Meet the editor

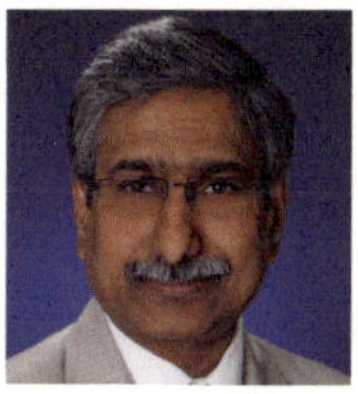

Mani T. Valarmathi is currently the Director of Research and Development at Religen Inc., a life science company in Pennsylvania, USA. He began his scientific career as a cancer geneticist, but soon became captivated by the emerging and translational fields of stem cell biology, tissue engineering, and regenerative medicine. After obtaining a bachelor's degree in Chemistry from the University of Madras, Chennai, Tamil Nadu, India, he obtained an MBBS in Medicine and Surgery and an MD in Pathology from the same university, as well as a Ph.D. in Medical Biotechnology from All-India Institute of Medical Sciences, New Delhi, India. Over the past two decades, he has had extensive experience in research on various types of stem cells, and his research work has been focused on creating bioengineered human 3D vascularized tissue constructs for implantation purposes. At present, much of his research is directed toward developing innovative molecular genetic testing for precision and genetic medicine. He is a member of many prestigious national and international professional societies and scientific organizations, including the International Society for Stem Cell Research (ISSCR), Tissue Engineering and Regenerative Medicine International Society (TERMIS), American Association for Cancer Research (AACR), American Society for Investigative Pathology (ASIP), American Society for Clinical Pathology (ASCP), American Chemical Society (ACS), European Society of Cardiology (ESC), International Society for Heart Research (ISHR), American Society of Gene & Cell Therapy (ASGCT), and American Heart Association (AHA).

Contents

Preface

Worldwide, breast cancer is the most common cancer among women, impacting more than 2 million women each year. It is the most common non-skin malignancy in women and the second leading cause of cancer death in women after lung cancer. Ovarian cancer is the eighth most commonly occurring cancer in women. The incidence of breast cancer varies greatly around the world, with more than 2.26 million new diagnoses made annually.

In Western societies, one in eight women is prone to develop breast cancer at some time in her life and some 15% to 20% of women with breast cancer have a positive family history of the disorder. Thus, it is expected that many families will experience more than one case because shared familial risk factors, for example, genes and environment, cause a greater incidence of cancer. Up to 20% of affected women have an affected first- or second-degree relative. Conceivably, many of these represent chance coincidences, but statistical analysis reveals that in 5% to 10% of women with breast cancer the condition is truly familial.

Mutations in the *BRCA1/2* genes are the most common cause of hereditary breast and ovarian cancer (HBOC), and HBOC is an autosomal dominant cancer predisposition syndrome. Individuals with HBOC have a high risk for breast and ovarian cancers and a moderate risk for other cancers, such as prostate, pancreatic, melanoma, and fallopian tube cancers. Nevertheless, not all individuals who inherit a mutation in *BRCA1/2* genes will eventually develop cancer (due to *reduced penetrance*), and the signs and symptoms, type, and age of cancer will also vary within families (due to *variable expressivity*).

Since both *BRCA1* and *BRCA2* genes have very large coding sequences and cancer susceptibility is a result of loss of function, the occurrence of pathogenic mutations might be anywhere in either one (*BRCA1* or *BRCA2*). As a result, genetic testing for *BRCA1/2* mutations is challenging and generally confined to individuals with a demonstrable strong family history or those belonging to certain high-risk ethnicity, for example, Ashkenazi Jewish and Icelandic, permitting easy DNA screening.

Two decades ago, my own doctoral research at the All-India Institute of Medical Sciences (AIIMS), New Delhi, resulted in the systematic discovery of numerous novel germline mutations in the *BRCA1* and *BRCA2* genes in Indian breast and/or breast-ovarian cancer families for the first time. In the Indian population, *BRCA* mutations are distributed throughout the coding sequence with no apparent clustering. Moreover, the study confirmed the strong influence of Ashkenazi Jewish founder mutation 185del AG (c.68_69delAG) in familial breast and/or ovarian cancer in Southern India. Thus, the identification of these novel mutations and the wider *BRCA* mutational spectrum ultimately led to the development of a mutation database for its program of *BRCA* genetic diagnostic testing and counseling in the Indian subcontinent. In this respect, I am deeply grateful to Dr. Abhilasha Agarwal for her cooperation and major contribution to the success of this work.

In recent years, there has been substantial development in *BRCA*-associated hereditary breast and/or breast-ovarian cancer research and its clinical applications, for instance, *BRCA* cancer biology and genomics, epidemiology and prevention, early detection and screening, and diagnosis and treatment. In addition, the advent of various emerging technologies, such as stem cell technology, genome editing technology, pharmacogenomics, and personalized medicine, and the knowledge gained from such studies, have not only enhanced our understanding of *BRCA*-associated cancer but also produced novel insights that could lead to the development and deployment of newer clinical/therapeutic interventions.

In this context, this book consolidates recent advances in *BRCA*-associated cancer biology and therapeutics, covering a broad spectrum of interrelated topics, and disseminates this essential knowledge in a comprehensible way to a scientific and clinical audience as well as patients, caregivers, and drug and device manufactures, especially to support breast cancer product development.

In this context, the ultimate purpose of this book is dispelling the existing classic mysteries of *BRCA* genes, for instance: (1) Why do *BRCA1* and *BRCA2* mutations lead to tumors in such a well-defined subset of human tissues? (2) Are breasts and ovary exposed to higher rates of DNA damage? (3) Do other tissues have a better back-up DNA repair system and, if so, what might that be? (4) Are these tissues less efficient at eliminating *BRCA*-deficient cells, enabling survival mutations to arise and tumors to form? (5) Finally, how can we take advantage of this deficiency in homologous recombination to specifically kill *BRCA*-mutant cells in cancer patients?

Written by leading experts in basic science and clinical care, this book consists of eight chapters over five sections. The **first section** provides an overview of HBOC syndrome. **Chapter 1** emphasizes the current challenges and future perspectives within the context of the advancement of genetic and precision medicine.

The **second section** deals with the history of *BRCA* discovery. **Chapter 2** depicts the initial steps that led to the discovery of *BRCA* genes using both genetic and statistical tools by diverse groups simultaneously, culminating in one of the best examples of how a scientific discovery may change human society for years to come.

The **third section** discusses the current understanding of *BRCA* structure and function. **Chapter 3** synthesizes the pleiotropic biological functions of both *BRCA1/2* genes and how their interactions with many other critical cellular proteins can contribute to various normal and abnormal cellular functions. It also discusses the clinical relevance of *BRCA* genes and how defects caused by *BRCA* gene mutations might be leveraged to develop newer targets for personalized medicine. **Chapter 4** examines *BRCA1*-associated RING domain-1 (*BARD1*) gene structure and its function in physiological and pathophysiological contexts, highlighting the dual function of the *BARD1* gene both as an oncogene and anti-oncogene, but also highlighting the epigenetic effect on *BARD1* gene expression and the biological consequence of it.

The **fourth section** explores *BRCA*-associated cancers, such as ovarian and prostate cancers. **Chapter 5** underscores the significance of *BRCA1/2* mutations in the development of prostate cancer and its increasing clinical significance with respect to metastatic and lethal prostate cancers. It crystallizes the essence of latest findings and the role of *BRCA* genes alterations pertaining to prostate cancer and emphasizes the importance of a detailed understanding of the complex DNA damage repair network in prostate cancer along with other unstable genomic alterations, providing deeper insights into the diverse functions of poly (adenosine diphosphate-ribose) polymerases (PARPs) and other potential contributors of synthetic lethality. **Chapter 6** provides a comprehensive view of the initiation and progression of ovarian cancer and delves deeper into various genetic and non-genetic factors that govern the ovarian epithelial cancers, with special emphasis on personalized medicine. It also examines why despite recent advancement, insights, and elucidation of various molecular mechanisms underpinning ovarian cancer development, advancement of efficacious therapy for ovarian carcinomas has been problematic, especially for the high-grade serous carcinomas.

The **fifth section** focuses on *BRCA* genetic testing, a tool to gain information, and genetic counselling, a process that helps interpret the information and place it in a personal context. **Chapter 7** delineates the prevalence of *BRCA1/2* mutations in Mexico, as well as the diagnostic and prognostic implication of founder mutations of *BRCA* in the Mexican population and its translation impact on routine clinical practice. **Chapter 8** addresses the most critical factors that govern the study of Quality of Life (QoL) in cancer patients, especially pertaining to *BRCA1/2* germline pathogenic variants and their relevance in cancer risk assessment, personalized medicine management, and cancer prevention. In addition, the chapter synthesizes the evolution of the evaluation of the QoL study according to the current needs of patients with *BRCA* mutations.

This book is a valuable resource not only for medical and allied health students but also for researchers, clinical and nurse geneticists, genetic counselors, and physician assistants. This quick reference will benefit anyone desiring thorough knowledge pertaining to recent advances in *BRCA*-related cancer biology and its associated diagnostic and therapeutic challenges.

I would like to thank the staff of IntechOpen who have produced this book so efficiently, particularly Author Service Manager Ana Javor and Commissioning Editor Marija Nezirović for providing excellent support throughout the preparation of this book. They were remarkably patient and persistent. Finally, this book is dedicated to the loving memory of my beloved parents, the light of a lantern.

Mani T. Valarmathi, MD, Ph.D.
Clinical Molecular Diagnostic Laboratory,
Religen Inc. | A Life Science Company,
Plymouth Meeting, Pennsylvania, USA

Section 1

Hereditary Breast and Ovarian Cancer Syndrome

Chapter 1

Introductory Chapter: The Influence of BRCA1/2 Genes Mutations on Hereditary Breast and Ovarian Cancer Syndrome - Is it in your Genes?

Mani T. Valarmathi

1. Introduction

Worldwide, breast cancer is even now the most common cancer among women, impacting over 2 million women each year, and still causes the maximum number of cancer-related deaths among women. The incidence of breast cancer varies greatly around the world, with over 2.26 million new diagnoses made annually. In 2022, in the United States (US), more than 287,000 women are expected to be newly diagnosed with the invasive breast cancer; in addition, about 51,400 new cases of ductal carcinoma *in situ* (DCIS) will be diagnosed. Overall, nearly 43,000 women are expected to die from the disease. Breast cancer is not only a women's disease, but over 2700 new cases of invasive breast cancer are also expected to be diagnosed in men in 2022, and nearly 500 men are expected to die from it. Moreover, it is estimated that there were more than 168,000 women living with metastatic breast cancer in the US in 2020 (most recent estimate available). Consequently, breast cancer is the most frequent cancer among women in the US, accounting for 31% of newly diagnosed cancers. Ovarian cancer is the eighth among all cancers, and only lung cancer kills more women and is the second most common cancer in women. Thus, invasive cancer of breast is the most common non-skin malignancy in women and is second only to lung cancer as cause of cancer deaths worldwide [1–5].

Breast cancer arises from the sequential accumulation of genetic (mutations or DNA alterations) and epigenetic changes, occurring over a span of years. Like other cancers, breast cancer is clonal proliferations that arise from cells with multiple genetic aberrations, acquisition of which is influenced by hormonal exposure and inherited susceptibility genes. Almost 12% of breast cancers occur due to inheritance of identifiable susceptibility gene or genes. The main known susceptibility genes for familial breast cancer are, for example, *BRCA1* (*BRCA1* DNA repair associated), *BRCA2* (*BRCA2* DNA repair associated), *TP53* (tumor protein p53), *CHEK2* (checkpoint kinase 2), and *PALB2* (partner and localizer of *BRCA2*). They are all tumor suppressor genes that are involved in ensuring the integrity of the genome. They are part of the systems that detect and repair DNA damage, and interact with many other critical cellular proteins, thus preventing the genomic instability. It is likely that complete inactivation of these tumor suppressor genes leads to loss of function of these proteins, resulting in a mutator phenotype, and consequently heightened propensity to accumulate genetic damage that enhances cancer development [6].

Everyone is at risk of breast cancer, the most important and strongest risk factors are estrogen stimulation (being born female) or age (getting older), and the risk of developing breast cancer is age dependent and increases with age. In the case of a man, the older a man is, the more likely he is to get breast cancer. However, breast cancer is much less common in men than in women. In the US, a woman in the general population has about a 1 in 8 chance (~13%) of being diagnosed during her lifetime. This also means that there is a 7 in 8 chance she will never have the disease. Similarly, a man's lifetime risk of breast cancer is about 1 in 833 (~0.1%). However, it is equally important to remember that the risk is highly dependent on age; for example, the chance of a women being diagnosed during her earlier life (30th year) is less than 1 in 204, whereas the chance of being diagnosed in her later life (70th year) is 1 in 24 [7]. Hence, unfortunately, of all the identified risk factors that can cause breast cancer, age is the major risk factor, the older the woman, the greater her risk [2, 5, 7].

A series of landmark discoveries during 1990 greatly enhanced our understanding of the role of genes in breast cancer. Currently, there exists a common consensus that around 10% of breast cancers arise mainly due to the influence of a disease-causing mutation with which the individual was born. The role of these putative genes that predispose women to breast cancer can be divided into three categories. For example, (i) the first category is a set of genes that so dramatically increase the lifetime risk, which can be presumed as causing an autosomal dominant disorder with "*incomplete penetrance*," that is because not all members harboring the mutation eventually develop the cancer; (ii) the second category is a set of potentially considerable "*low penetrance*" genes that increase the risk, but not to the level that families in which they are found stand out as breast cancer families; and finally, (iii) the third group is a set of "*very rare single-gene disorders*" that includes breast cancer as a feature, which represents for only about 1% of all breast cancers [5–6].

2. *BRCA1* and *BRCA2* genes

In 1990, linkage analysis in a large collection of multicase families (studies of early-onset or premenopausal breast cancer) pinpointed a possible susceptibility locus for early-onset or premenopausal breast cancer at chromosome 17q21, eventually leading to identification of the *BRCA1* gene. Since a proportion of families with early-onset breast cancer did not demonstrate linkage to this region, a further round of systematic analysis in *BRCA1*-negative families revealed linkage to chromosome 13q12.3, resulting in the identification of *BRCA2* gene [6].

In western societies since 1 woman in 8 is prone to develop breast cancer at some time in her life, and some 15 to 20% of women with breast cancer have a positive family history of the disorder, it is expected that many families have more than one case—when shared familial risk factors, for example, genes and environment, cause a higher incidence of cancer. Up to 20% of affected women have an affected first- or second-degree relative. Conceivably, many of these represent chance coincidences, but statistical analysis reveals that in 5 to 10% of women with breast cancer the condition is truly familial (hereditary, due to a single-gene mutation). However, in earlier studies using a biased set of families for a *BRCA1/2* mutation carrier, the initial estimates of risk have been variously estimated between 60% and 85%. The population-based survey shows lower risk [2, 4–6].

In addition to the risk to the female relative is greater when one or more of the following factors is present that is, at high risk for hereditary breast and ovarian cancer (HBOC): the markers of *BRCA1/2* mutations include the following: (i) a cluster of cases in close female relatives; (ii) cases with unusually early onset (early age [>35–45 years] at presentation, both invasive and DCIS); (iii) bilateral cases (the occurrence of bilateral disease); (iv) families with both breast and ovarian cancers—particularly a feature with *BRCA1* variants (the occurrence of ovarian cancer, epithelial); and (v) cases with male breast cancer—particularly a feature with *BRCA2* variants (a paternal [or close male relative] history of breast cancer). However, none of these features is entirely specific to *BRCA1/2* breast cancer [8–11].

In general, mutations in *BRCA1* and *BRCA2* are responsible for 80–90% of "*single-gene*" familial breast cancers and about 3% of all breast cancers. Penetrance (*the percentage of carriers who develop breast cancer*) varies from 30 to 90% depending upon the specific mutation present. In women, considering the general population, breast and ovarian cancer risks are 1 in 8 (~13%) and 1 in 50 (~2%), respectively, the *BRCA1/2* genes clearly carry a significantly elevated risk. Equally, the risk of breast and prostate cancer in population of men are ~0.1% and ~ 14%, respectively. Mutations in the *BRCA1/2* genes are the most common cause of HBOC, and HBOC is an autosomal dominant cancer predisposition syndrome. Individuals with HBOC have high-risk for breast and ovarian cancers and moderate risk for other cancers, such as prostate, pancreatic, melanoma, and fallopian tube. Nevertheless, not all individuals who inherit a mutation in *BRCA1/2* genes will eventually develop cancer (due to *reduce penetrance*), and the signs and symptoms, type, and age of cancer will vary within families due to *variable expressivity* [1–5].

Pathogenic variants in *BRCA1* and *BRCA2* account for nearly 15% of cases of familial breast cancer. The lifetime risk of developing the disease is 60–90%, in case of carriers of disease-causing *BRCA1* variants, as well as a 40–60% lifetime risk of developing an ovarian cancer. Similarly, the carriers of pathogenic *BRCA2* variants have a 45–85% lifetime risk of developing breast cancer and confer a slightly lower risk of 10–30% for ovarian cancer. In addition, male breast cancer risk is elevated in

Type of Cancer	**Women**			**Men**		
	***BRCA1* Carrier**	***BRCA2* Carrier**	**General Population**	***BRCA1* Carrier**	***BRCA2* Carrier**	**General Population**
Breast cancer	60–90%	45–85%	13%	1–5%	7–8%	0.1%
Ovarian cancer	40–60%	10–30%	2%	—	—	—
Prostate cancer	—	—	—	*	~15–25%	14%
Pancreatic cancer	2–3%	3–5%	1%	2–3%	3–5%	1%
Melanoma	**	3–5%	1–2%	**	3–5%	1–2%

BRCA—Breast cancer susceptibility genes.
**Overall increased lifetime risk but no convincing evidence, BRCA1 carriers may develop early-onset prostate cancer.*
***Not well defined or no known increased cancer risk.*

Table 1.
Lifetime cancer risks (by age 70) for BRCA mutation carriers in comparison to the general population.

carriers of *BRCA1/2* mutations (7 to 8%), although it is higher in *BRCA2* gene carriers, and the lifetime risk of developing prostate cancer is around 20%, in the case of male *BRCA2* gene carriers (**Table 1**) [5–6].

The remaining known susceptibility genes, such as *TP53* (17p13.1) and *CHEK2* (22q12.1), account for less than 10% of familial breast cancers. Collectively, germline mutations in *TP53* (Li-Fraumeni syndrome) and mutations in *CHEK2* (confers modest, rather than high risk) account for about 8% of breast cancer and are caused by single-gene defects. Besides, *TP53* is the most frequently mutated gene in sporadic breast cancers (non-germline or somatic). The other genes that play a part in hereditary breast cancer, for instance *PALB2,* which is associated with a 30–60% lifetime risk of breast cancer. Most of these genes control checkpoints in the cell cycle and thus could influence cell division; after DNA damage, p53 and *CHEK2* induce cell cycle arrest and either repair their DNA or die by apoptosis, thus playing complex and interrelated roles in maintaining the genomic integrity [6].

Since both *BRCA1* and *BRCA2* genes have very large coding sequences and considering the fact that cancer susceptibility is a result of loss of function, so the occurrence of pathogenic mutations might be anywhere in either one (BRCA1 or BRCA2); as a result, genetic testing for *BRCA1/2* mutations is challenging and generally confined to individuals with a demonstrable strong family history or those belonging to certain high-risk ethnicity, for example, Ashkenazi Jewish and Icelandic. An estimated frequency of about 1 in 40 Ashkenazi Jews carries a *BRCA* mutation, a prevalence about threefold greater than the background. Three founder variants—185delAG (c.68_69delAG), 5382insC (c.5266dupC), and 6174delT (c.594delT)—are very frequent in Ashkenazi Jewish population, permitting easy DNA screening. However, negative screen does not exclude other *BRCA* variants or a variant in another high- and/or moderate-risk gene. Similarly, other populations, such as Icelanders, French-Canadians, and Pakistanis, also have their own specific founder mutations [6–11].

3. Concluding remarks and perspectives

Inherited cancer susceptibility syndromes (ICSS), such as HBOC, are caused by genetic mutations that place patients at an increased risk of developing cancer. These cancer-predisposing syndromes carry a risk of an additional primary tumor (bilateral or multifocal in the case of breast cancer) and clinically appear at a relatively young age compared with sporadic breast cancers. The tumors may occur at a variety of sites in the body; however, in most cases, one type of cancer predominates. The ultimate goal of screening individuals at high risk of familial cancer is either prevention (such as a change in lifestyle or diet) or early detection of cancer. The identification of *BRCA* carriers is important since increased surveillance, drug therapy (chemoprevention), and prophylactic surgery (risk-reducing surgeries, such as mastectomy and/or salpingo-oophorectomy) can reduce cancer-related morbidity and mortality.

Author details

Mani T. Valarmathi
Clinical Molecular Diagnostic Laboratory, Religen Inc. – A Life Science Company, Plymouth Meeting, Pennsylvania, USA

*Address all correspondence to: valarmathi64@hotmail.com

References

[1] World Cancer Research Fund International. Cancer Trends: Worldwide Cancer Data. London, UK: World Cancer Research Fund International; 2020

[2] The Susan G. Komen Breast Cancer Foundation. Breast Cancer Information. Dallas, TX: The Susan G

[3] Ferlay J, Ervik M, Lam F, Colombet M, Mery L, Piñeros M, et al. Global Cancer Observatory: Cancer Today. Lyon, France: International Agency for Research on Cancer; 2020

[4] American Cancer Society. Breast Cancer Facts & Figures 2022. Atlanta, GA: American Cancer Society; 2022

[5] Moyer VA. Risk assessment, genetic counselling, and genetic testing for *BRCA*-related cancer in women: U.S. preventive services task force recommendation statement. Annals of Internal Medicine. 2014;**160**:271-281. DOI: 10.7326/M13-2747

[6] Read A, Donnai D. New Clinical Genetics. 4th ed. UK: Scion Publishing Limited; 2021. pp. 175-206

[7] Howlader N, Noone AM, Krapcho M, Miller D, Brest A, Yu M, et al., editors. SEER Cancer Statistics Review, 1975-2017. Bethesda, MD: National Cancer Institute; 2020

[8] Valarmathi MT, Agarwal A, Deo SS, Shukla NK, Das SN. *BRCA1* germline mutations in Indian familial breast cancer. Human Mutation. 2003 Jan;**21**(1):98-99. DOI: 10.1002/humu.9099

[9] Valarmathi MT, Sawhney M, Deo SS, Shukla NK, Das SN. Novel germline mutations in the *BRCA1* and *BRCA2* genes in Indian breast and breast-ovarian cancer families. Human Mutation. 2004;**23**(2):205. DOI: 10.1002/humu.9213

[10] Welsch PL, King MC. *BRCA1* and *BRCA2* and the genetics of breast and ovarian cancer. Human Molecular Genetics. 2001;**10**(7):705-713. DOI: 10.1093/hmg/10.7.705

[11] Wooster R, Weber BL. Breast and ovarian cancer. The New England Journal of Medicine. 2003;**348**(23):2339-2347. DOI: 10.1056/NEJMra012284

Section 2

BRCA Discovery

Chapter 2

Discovery of BRCA Mutations: Historical Perspective of Its Scientific, Clinical and Social Impact

Natalia B. Burachik, Ana Laura Ortiz and Edith C. Kordon

Abstract

In the human genome, BRCA1 and BRCA2 (for **BR**east **CA**ncer 1 and 2) genes encode for proteins involved in several functions that are crucial for the maintenance of genome stability and integrity. They participate in DNA damage response and repair pathways and, therefore, act as tumor suppressor genes. Mutations in these genes, which are located in chromosomes 17q21 and 13q13 respectively, are responsible for a great fraction of inherited breast and ovarian cancers, as well as other pathologies, such as Fanconi Anemia. Approximately 30 years ago, a report from a group of the School of Public Health at the University of California about a hypothetical gene that led to predisposition to early-onset breast cancer in certain families changed the history of breast cancer research, diagnosis, and prevention. Nowadays, the accessibility of genetic testing and the availability of different approaches as wide coverage screenings, prophylactic mastectomies, and risk-lowering drugs benefits BRCA1 and BRCA2 mutation carriers enormously. This chapter summarizes the unique trajectory of BRCA research and its scientific and social implications.

Keywords: history, BRCA1, BRCA2, breast cancer, ovarian cancer

1. Introduction

Breast cancer is the world's most prevalent cancer type. In 2020, 2.3 million women were diagnosed with breast cancer and 685.000 deaths were reported globally, ranking as the most common cause of cancer death among women [1]. From the 1930s to the 1970s breast cancer mortality rate remained quite constant, but since 1980, thanks to the implementation of early detection procedures, there has been notable progress in survival rates. Nowadays, some risk factors that lead to breast cancer are well identified and, in general, the population is better aware about them, as the information became more available in the era of digital communication. However, this progress has not been even among different regions in the world. Data suggest that the low income countries have diminished survival rates due to less access to information and early testing [2].

The high rates of breast cancer incidence and mortality in women of certain families led to a long search for the causes of inherent susceptibility to develop this illness. Around 1970, a global race to discover those factors started and reached the first milestone in 1994 that was the Science publication reporting BRCA1 sequencing, which was soon followed by the discovery and sequencing of a second gene, BRCA2. This chase indelibly marked the cancer and genetic research fields, but also labeled the initiation of the ongoing discussion about the role of private companies on gene discovery and patenting. Since then, medical progress based on gene and mutation discoveries have involved not only scientific, but also major ethical and commercial debates. Now, almost 30 years later, those issues are still controversial. In addition, and in spite of the huge advance of basic knowledge about those genes, several fundamental questions remain unanswered, such as why, in people carrying a mutated BRCA gene copy, hormone-sensitive tissues are the most prone to neoplastic transformation. In this chapter, we will focus on these topics, which are still under debate.

2. Historical aspects about the discovery and diagnostic usage of BRCA1 and BRCA2 mutations

In December of 1990, Mary Claire King's group published a research article reporting the analysis they performed in 23 extended families with a very high incidence of early-onset breast cancer. Analyzed cases were chosen meticulously according to their pathology records. Using different polymorphic markers and four statistical approaches, they associated those tumors with alterations in chromosome 17q21 [3]. Is important to underscore that only the position was then reported, and without the complete human genome sequenced, the gene that caused early-onset breast cancer was merely hypothetical. Then, the "race" to specifically establish the mutated gene responsible for hereditary breast cancer syndrome began.

A year later, Gilbert M. Lenoir and his colleagues confirmed King's team finding, but also associated that chromosomal location to a proportion of hereditary ovarian cancers [4] and Mary Claire King named this still hypothetical gene BReast CAncer 1 (BRCA1). In 1992, King's group reduced the previously located area to a 8-cM region that was very likely to include this gene. They pointed out that it would be a mistake to oversimplify and consider that mutated BRCA1 was involved in breast cancer initiation in the general population, since the analyzed cases corresponded specifically not only to families with high breast cancer incidence, but also to patients with early-onset disease. In addition, they indicated that the data that linked the breast cancer syndrome to chromosome 17q was heterogenous, suggesting that it might be another gene involved in the development of familial breast cancer, and/or associated to a high frequency of sporadic cases in older-onset families. Importantly, they also reported that it was not possible to distinguish sporadic to familial breast cancer by clinical criteria. Therefore, the involvement of BRCA1 in the inherited risk of mammary tumor development was solely defined by the identification of mutations in breast cancer patients of susceptible families [5].

It was not until October 1994, that the predicted amino acid sequences of BRCA1 and some probable predisposing mutations were published by Mark Skolnick *et al* in *Science* [6]. Up to that time, King's laboratory as well as other groups were close but not able to sequence the whole gene, yet they were later responsible for identifying several different mutations in affected families. Importantly, a month earlier that same year (September 1994) the BRCA2 gene was identified in chromosome 13q through a similar strategy to the previously used, but analyzing 15 families with multiple cases of early-onset breast cancer not linked to BRCA1. Interestingly, men bearing BRCA2 mutations showed higher breast cancer risk, but women had less chances to develop ovarian tumors than BRCA1 mutation carriers [7]. The following year, *Nature* published the BRCA2 predicted amino acid sequence as well as this gene mutations based on the Human Genome Project as well as data provided by the Sanger Center and Washington University [8].

Localization and sequencing of the BRCA genes did not provide any clue about the possible biological roles of the proteins encoded by them. They neither showed homologies to any other protein characterized up to that date, nor distinguishable functional domains. Therefore, it was not rapidily elucidated which were BRCA1 and BRCA2 biological roles and whether they overlapped totally or partially. Although the proteins are not similar in their primary sequences, they share several particular features. For example, both are surprisingly large and highly charged, and the corresponding genes have many exons, which suffer alternative splicing. Interestingly, exon 11, where the interactive regions with RAD51 are located, is particularly large and encodes about half a protein in both cases. Curiously, if not for the classic genetic approach to detect them, neither BRCA nor BRCA2 would have been selected as tumor suppressor candidates for to the information provided by their sequences.

The data that arose soon after their discovery were mostly related to the impact of different BRCA1 and BRCA2 mutations on cancer risk. It was determined that some subpopulations with a high tendency to develop breast cancer carried alternative genetic variants in their germline and that the prevalent mutations had been established as a consequence of a founder effect. This happens when a small group of people remains separated from the original population and, after several generations of interbreeding, rare mutations present in the first generation become more frequent. For example, Ashkenazi Jew families, whose ancestors lived in Central and Eastern Europe, are particularly affected by three well-known founder mutations; BRCA1-185delAG, 5382insC, and BRCA2-6174delT, with an overall rate of 2.6% (1/40), in contrast to the 0.2% (1/500) of these three BRCA1/2 mutation carriers in the general population [9]. Other founder mutations have been determined in various European populations, such as some Norwegian, Dutch, and Icelandic families [9, 10]. The possibility of having information about large numbers of people with the same mutation opened the door to analyze the penetrance of such variants, together with the importance of risk-modifying factors that could affect the outcome of the disease [9].

By the age of 70, women who carry a BRCA1 or a BRCA2 clinically relevant mutation, have a 50–65% or 50–55% chance, respectively, of developing breast cancer, while that probability goes down to 7% for women without any of those mutations. In the case of ovarian cancer, the risk is between 35 and 70% for women with a BRCA1 gene mutation, it is lower (10–30%) for those who bear a BRCA2 mutation, but less than 2% for women who do not have any of those variants [11]. For men, only BRCA2 mutation carriers have a significantly higher risk of developing breast or prostate cancer. However, all people who possess one BRCA1 or BRCA2 mutation have an increased risk of developing pancreatic cancer and Fanconi anemia. An increased susceptibility to melanoma has been observed only in the case of BRCA2 inherited gene mutations [12]. It is important to remember that BRCA mutations can also occur sporadically.

BRCA1/2 mutation carriers have between 40 to 80% more chances of getting a second primary contralateral breast tumor. However, it is remarkable that not all women carrying a BRCA1 or BRCA2 mutation get breast cancer. Therefore, there are other risk factors involved in the occurrence of this illness, even for women who inherit the harmful mutations. Interestingly, BRCA1 and BRCA2 female carriers tend to develop different breast cancer subtypes. The first are more likely to have triple-negative tumors (*i.e.* Estrogen receptor-negative, Progesterone receptor-negative, and HER2-negative), which do not have specific clinically successful treatments, while the latter show a higher probability to develop estrogen receptor-positive (*i.e.* luminal) breast cancer, that usually receive endocrine therapy [11].

Even though most breast cancers do not involve a specific hereditary component, in particular cases it is recommended to take a genetic test in order to find out whether BRCA1 or BRCA2 is mutated in the germ line [11]. This analysis (patented on 1997 in the US) and owned by Myriad Genetics until 2013, is commonly recommended only under certain conditions, such as high incidence of breast or ovarian cancer in the family, belonging to certain ancestries (*i.e.* Ashkenazi Jew), etc. Nonetheless, until 2013, a critical aspect for which the test was not massively advised was the price, which was over US$3000. Undeniably, a value not accessible to everyone. In addition, there were many other elements that the clinicians took into account before prescribing the BRCA1/2 genetic test, as the psychological impact of the result on the patient and their family as well as her/his predisposition to undergo prophylactic measures.

Almost from the beginning, it was clear that gene testing was not the magic answer to all clinical questions. In 1997, a review article clearly showed the problems associated with gene testing, which can be summarized into two main points intrinsically related: one related to technical and biological issues and the other associated to understanding and usefulness. Specifically, for the detection of BRCA 1/2 mutations, technology available in the late 90s was still slow, expensive and not too sensitive. In addition, there were variants still unknown and/or with no existing information about its biological association with cancer [13]. Genetic testing carries complex issues that even today are misunderstood by the general public and health professionals, so it is necessary to provide the required knowledge to both. Otherwise, gene testing may result useless, cause a waste of resources and be dangerously utilized.

The result of the gene test can be positive, negative, or indicate a variant of uncertain significance (VUS, when the harmfulness of the detected mutation is unknown). If a known variant is found, their relatives can be tested to determine whether they carry the same mutation, which is less expensive than sequencing the whole gene for each of them. In many cases, health insurance covers BRCA testing if the person meets the established criteria. With an accurate diagnosis and treatment at an early stage, women who have a BRCA1/2 inherited gene mutation present a similar survival rate than those who develop breast cancer without an inherent genetic component [10, 11]. In recent years, the recommendation of testing based only on familial high cancer incidence has been questioned. According to a report published in 2015, half the breast cancer patients with BRCA1/2 mutations did not meet family history criteria for testing, so they learned they were carriers after cancer had already developed. This was a breaking point in cancer prevention and, based on those and other similar results, some researchers and clinicians encourage population screenings that enable a much more complete and cost-effective identification of carriers [14].

In a study carried in 1999, among 200 women with breast and/or ovarian cancer, who were offered testing for BRCA1 and BRCA2 free of charge, a high proportion of them had overestimated their risk of having a mutation, and some of them faced difficulties with their health insurance if the outcome of their analysis resulted positive [15]. These facts reflect how the lack of general knowledge about genetics, and particularly, cancer genetics may lead to unnecessary psychological stress, and the economical and social pressure suffered by who is (or suspects to be) a BRCA1/2 mutation carrier. A boom of testing occurred right after May 2013, when Angelina Jolie shared her breast cancer family history in the *New York Times* [16]. In an opinion article, the well-known actress and director, announced that upon learning that she carried a BRCA1 mutation, she decided to undergo double mastectomy to reduce her risk of dying from cancer. Later, she also had her ovaries and fallopian tubes removed. In that commentary, she encouraged women to take a genetic test if they believed they were highly susceptible to develop breast and/or ovarian cancer and, in that way, to take active action to prevent the onset and progression of these diseases. According to doctors and medical centers, this event significantly increased BRCA testing and public interest in this subject, a phenomenon baptized by the media as the "Angelina Jolie effect" [17].

There are different options for BRCA1/2 mutation carriers to decrease cancer risk, such as taking early detection tests and/or undergoing surgeries, like prophylactic mastectomy or oophorectomy (or both). When the first women diagnosed with those genetic variants had to make a decision, the data on the long term outcome of these procedures were very limited. Nevertheless, many social and clinical studies about their efficacy have taken place since then. In 1997, a special report showed that prophylactic mastectomy led to a higher increase in life expectancy than prophylactic oophorectomy, but there were much better benefits when both procedures were done [18, 19]. On the other hand, the advantages of those procedures tended to decrease with increasing age, being almost not significant at all when they were performed in women over 60 years old. That is why BRCA1/2 mutation testing is recommended for women under that age [19].

Some women may avoid BRCA testing for fear of the adverse effects of prevention treatments if they resulted positive. Breast and/or ovaries removal may affect them physically and emotionally as it may lead to fertility problems and issues with their body image. Oophorectomy causes early menopause, which can induce weight gain, an increased risk of cardiovascular diseases, osteoporosis and sexual discomfort. In addition, tamoxifen and raloxifene tratments have rare but severe side effects, such as uterine cancer, blood clots, and stroke [17]. Therefore, precise and early advice about pros and cons of these preventive approaches is required so candidates for these procedures can choose what is best for themselves [19].

Presently, prophylactic mastectomy can reduce the risk of breast cancer by over 90%, but for those who do not want to go through surgery, it is advisable to take a yearly screening with breast magnetic resonance imaging (MRI) (or mammography, which is less recommended because a harmful BRCA variant might be particularly sensitive to the DNA-damaging effects of radiation), as well as biannual pelvic ultrasonography and cancer antigen 125 (CA-125) testing. Noteworthy this protein has been identified in women with advanced ovarian cancer, but it has not been found in early stages of this illness, therefore screening based on its detection has not improved survival [10].

BRCA1/2 deficient cells may be sensible to classic chemotherapeutic drugs that arrest replication and DNA cross-linking agents, like those based on platinum components. Therefore, these drugs, may be recommended to mutation carriers [20]. Since normal BRCA1 protein participates in DNA repair mechanisms by homologous recombination, in the past few years, new drugs (like olaparib and talazoparib), which inhibit PARP1 enzyme and therefore block DNA reparation pathway by base excision repair, have been developed. These drugs leave a gap in the single strand

DNA that arrest the replication fork and convert the single strand break into a double strand break. This leads to cell death in cells whose repair mechanisms by homologous recombination are damaged because of BRCA1 function failure. Currently, there are four PARP inhibitors approved for clinical use, although it is essential to continue investigating possible new synthetic therapeutic and lethal targets, because PARP inhibitors have toxic effects on normal cells and some tumor cells may be resistant to these treatments [20, 21].

Shortly after BRCA1 sequencing was completed, Myriad Genetics, a biotechnology and molecular diagnostic company founded in 1991 in the US, requested patents over BRCA1 gene and over BRCA2 later on. They were granted in 1997 for the US, in 2000 for Canada and in 2001 for Europe, obtaining seven patents in total. In the country or countries where an invention has been patented, their owners control its making, using, and selling for a specific period, which, in the case of BRCAs, corresponded to twenty years. Laws of nature, physical phenomena and abstract ideas are not patentable. However, the BRCA applications were granted because the US Patent and Trademark Office (USPTO) argued that isolated human gene sequences were patentable because human labor was needed to extract and purify them. Noteworthy, a similar stance was taken by the European Union.

BRCA1 patent provided Myriad Genetics the rights over the diagnostic or therapeutic use of this gene, whatever technique was utilized for carry on the assays, as well as all mutations found in familial breast and ovarian cancers, and their usage for determining cancer predisposition. Similarly, BRCA2 most frequent allelic variants, identified mutations associated to disease and methods for determining nucleotide sequence variations were protected [22]. Therefore, Myriad had a wide span of patent rights that provided them the monopoly for BRCA testing [23]. The company required all laboratories to send the DNA samples to Myriad headquarters in Salt Lake City, Utah for testing. That involved an initial cost of 1600 US$ and they could decide what research might be carried out on those genes, by whom and how much any resulting therapy or diagnostic test would cost [24]. This arrangement, which also included complete control over any further research on the diagnosis of certain breast tumors, was unprecedented in the field of genetic testing [22]. Furthermore, Myriad promoted the BRCA test to physicians and to the general US population on TV and print media, causing unnecessary anxiety about breast cancer risk [25]. In September 2007, the company released a questionable direct-to-consumer (DTC) marketing campaign offering genetic testing for 3100 US$ without requiring personal medical advice for its solicitation. Noteworthy, the prices were increased while new technology actually made testing less expensive [26]. However, many laboratories performed diagnostic BRCA1/2 tests without observing patenting rights, putting themselves at risk of being sued.

With the aim of canceling Myriad patents, many plaintiffs coaligned across different countries. Europe was the first to invalidate the BRCA patents with different arguments, including the Art. 52 (4) of the European Patent Convention: "Methods for treatment of the human or animal body by surgery or therapy and diagnostic methods practiced on the human or animal body shall not be regarded as inventions ..." and focusing on three points: Firstly, the lack of priority and absence of novelty, because gene sequences were already available in public databases when the third patent, which covered a specific set of mutations related to familial breast and ovarian cancer and their use in methods for determining predisposition for breast and/or ovarian cancer, was filed; secondly, the lack of inventiveness, for the same reasons indicated above, and thirdly because therapeutic uses of mutation sequences, in particular gene therapy methods, were not sufficiently described for implementing them effectively. Also, by 2002, the Institut Curie demonstrated that the methods used by Myriad Genetics to detect mutations, failed to identify about 10-20% of all expected mutations [22, 23]. In addition, Dr. Mary Clair King's article in JAMA proving that Myriad's tests missed a significant number of mutations, discredit this company and its rights on BRCA1/2 in the UK and Canada. In the US, the news were mainly covered by Utah from the perspective of Myriad, who rebutted the claim [27].

In 2010, a US District Court stated that all BRCA patent claims were invalid and that isolated DNA is 'not patentable subject matter'. Then, in 2011, the US Court of Appeals for the Federal Circuit overturned this ruling (2 to 1 decision); but in 2013, the Supreme Court decided to re-examine the lower courts' decisions and to analyze the claims on gene patenting [28]. Finally, the Supreme Court agreed with the plaintiffs that isolated gene sequences were not patentable because they were not "markedly different" from gene sequences already existing in nature [29].

With the expiration and overturning of BRCA patents, there were no more limitations on the offering of commercial testing. Also, these legal changes occurred approximately at the same time as the widespread adoption of massively parallel sequencing (MPS) technology, which allowed less expensive testing panels featured in turn-around times (TAT) [30].

At this point, we would like to go back to the woman behind this ongoing story, Mary-Claire King, whose contributions for society exceed the discovery of the BRCA genes. Born in 1946 in the US, she attended college and got a degree in mathematics inspired by two of her high-school teachers. Then, she went to the University of Berkeley for graduate school, where she took a genetics course and decided to follow that path. It was the 60s and a lot of social and political situations were taking place all over the world, and the States were not the exception. King was involved in social justice causes like the civil rights movement, and subsequently the anti-war movement. For her Ph.D. Thesis, mentored by Allan Wilson, one of the firsts to approach evolution from a molecular perspective, she demonstrated that humans and chimpanzees share 99% of their coding sequences [31], which caused an evolution revolution at that time.

In the early 1970s, Dr. King moved to South America with her husband in an exchange program between the University of California and the University of Chile. She taught genetics, statistics, and evolution until 1973, when a military coup overthrew President Allende's government. They could not stay, so the couple decided to return to the US. Back then, postdoc positions did not quite exist in academia, but as she said in a conversation with Ushma S. Neill, "*there were many jobs available in cancer research, because President Nixon had just launched the war on cancer. One of those jobs was at UCSF with a lovely pediatric oncologist named Nicholas Petrakis who had become interested in breast cancer*" [32]. Petrakis soon became her post-doc mentor and she started studying an inherited genetic component in breast cancer.

She obtained that position thanks to affirmative action, a policy aimed to balance gender inequality, a fact she noted in more than one interview. Her involvement in social justice was not only about her feminist position, but also her scientific collaboration in the investigation of human rights abuse. In the early 1980s, Dr. Cavalli-Sforza from Stanford, started teaching Dr. King, molecular genetics. And by that time, the Committee on Scientific Freedom and Responsibility of the American Association of Advancement of Science (AAAS), contacted him as a consultant for a genetic issue. In 1977, the Grandmothers of Plaza de Mayo (the "Abuelas", as they are commonly known in Argentina) had organized themselves in Buenos Aires during the last civil-military dictatorship, to demand the return of their grandchildren, who were born during the captivity of their missing ("desaparecidas") daughters. The "Abuelas" obtained good anecdotal evidence from some survivors and other witnesses about how those babies were given to different families. Then, they correctly proposed that it should be possible to establish the biological familial link by DNA comparison of the grandparents with their putative grandchildren, even if the parents were missing and presumed dead. To reach that goal, Dr. King and her colleagues created a genetic test that provided an "index of grandpaternity" ("índice de abuelitud"). Dr. King (who was fluent in Spanish) traveled to Buenos Aires to put the grandpaternity test into practice in June 1984, and that is how it began a 30-year collaboration with the organization of "Abuelas de Plaza de Mayo" [32–34]. Since then, and thank to that test, 130 grandchildren have been found by their biological families. Presently, Dr. King keeps on working at the University of Washington, trying to solve hereditary cases of breast cancer that cannot be explained by BRCA1 or BRCA2, but rather cryptic mutations that remain elusive [35].

2.1 Understanding the biological role of the Breast Cancer genes

The early reported BRCA1 and BRCA2 mutations coded for truncated proteins, and the loss of the wild-type allele (loss of heterozygosity, LOH) was detected in tumor samples from affected families [36]. The scientific community agreed on these genes being tumor suppressors, although the nucleotide sequences revealed nothing about their protein function. Starting in 1996, different groups around the world dedicated their efforts to decode the cellular localization and biological role of the BRCA proteins, because the first step to figure out how their deregulation could lead to disease was to understand their activities in physiological conditions.

Mouse models revealed that BRCA1 and BRCA2 were required for embryonic cellular proliferation, as different homozygous mutations resulted in embryonic lethality. The KO embryos showed no increased apoptosis, but cell proliferation was impaired and strong upregulation of the cell cycle regulator p21 was observed. In contrast, mouse with heterozygous mutations were phenotypically normal and fertile up to almost one year of age, although it was not ruled out the possibility of tumors may develop at more advanced age. The similarities displayed by embryos with homozygous null alleles for either BRCA1 or BRCA2 led to think that both genes acted in the same pathway during embryogenesis [37, 38].

BRCA1 and BRCA2 showed an incredibly similar pattern of expression through cell cycle when studied in normal and tumor-derived breast epithelial cells [39]. In synchronized cultured cells, gene expression reached a maximum in late-G1 and S-phase, suggesting a role for both genes in cell proliferation and cell cycle checkpoints. Soon, the first clue that BRCA1 and BRCA2 were actually involved in the DNA repair and homologous recombination came from the observation of co-localization and co-immunoprecipitation of BRCA1 with human Rad51 (hsRad51) in cultured cells [40]. However, it was then determined that it is BRCA2 the one that directly binds to hsRad51, while the interaction with BRCA1 would be indirect, requiring the participation of at least another protein [41]. hsRad51 is the human homolog of *E. coli* RecA and Rad51 in *Saccharomyces cerevisiae*, which are involved in DNA recombination and damage repair. In mouse and mammalian cells, homozygous knock-out of Rad51 displayed a very similar phenotype to BRCA1−/− and BRCA2 −/− mice, indicating the involvement of that protein in cell viability [42].

It has been shown that BRCA1 and BRCA2 colocalize in nuclear foci of somatic cells as a biochemical complex. In addition, these proteins also coincides with hRAD51 in DNA replication sites after exposure to damaging agents [43]. Furthermore, mouse cells with truncated *Brca2* gene have shown not only G1/S and G2 phase arrest, but also aberrant chromosomal number and structure [44]. Interestingly, cell cycle checkpoints and apoptosis mechanisms displayed no alterations [44]. These reports reinforced the idea that BRCA1 and BRCA2 share some common roles, acting coordinately to preserve chromosome stability. However, there must be functional differences between them that would account for the observed variation in cancer risk for BRCA1 and BRCA2 mutation carriers.

In 1996 and 1997 it was reported that both BRCA1 and BRCA2 contained domains that, when associated with the DNA-binding domain GAL4, induced transcriptional activation in yeast [45, 46]. Moreover, it has also been demonstrated that full-length BRCA1 was a component of the RNA Pol II holoenzyme [47]. Therefore, it has been proposed that the BRCAs may participate in transcription regulation. However, it has not been determined yet whether this activity would be independent from the DNA repair function. In addition, it also remains to be solved why mutation in genes coding proteins involved in very basic activities, such as DNA repair, required in every single cell type, induce high cancer risk only in very specific tissues. To date, there is still no right answer to this question. There are different theories about tissue-specific carcinogenesis caused mostly by BRCA1, but also BRCA2, in mutation carriers. The analysis and implications of this open question exceed the purpose of this chapter, but we briefly report here the leading hypothesis on this subject.

Based on certain BRCA deletion mutations found in cancer patients, it has been proposed that tissue specific carcinogenicity would be due to the loss of "breast-cancer cluster" regions (BCCRs) and "ovarian cancer cluster" regions (OCCRs) that are present in both *BRCA1* and *BRCA2* genes. Nevertheless, this proposition should be taken cautiously, because deletions in the proposed sequences would not only eliminate downstream exons coding for protein regions, but also might repress protein expression through nonsense-mediated mRNA decay. Therefore, those mutations, specifically those corresponding to the first few hundred nucleotides of the *BRCA1* or *BRCA2* coding sequences, would probably result into functionally "null" alleles, which should not cause tissue-specific effects [48]. Alternatively, it has been postulated that the higher cancer susceptibility of Estrogen-dependent organs to BRCA mutations would be due to the genotoxic effect that this hormone may exert on cells. Then, it has been suggested that hormone-responsive tissues might be particularly sensible to the failure of DNA damage reparation exerted by BRCA proteins [49]. On the other hand, another theory is based on the accumulation of R-loops, DNA–RNA hybrids, necessary for the differentiation of normal mammary luminal epithelial cells. In brief, BRCAs would be required for recruitment of some molecules involved in transcription (*i.e.* BRCA2 is necessary for PAF1 activity) and, in the absence of BRCA proteins chromatin disassembly may decrease. Then, transcription elongation would be obstructed causing accumulation of RNAPII in promoter-proximal pausing (PPP) sites generating R-loops which would lead to DNA breaks and consequently to genomic instability [50]. Growing evidence indicates the connection between R-loops and estrogen activity. These reports point out that genomic instability, increased in the scenario of BRCA1 or BRCA2 mutations, may be especially enhanced in estrogen-responsive tissues such as the breast [51]. This establishes another possible explanation for the high risk of BRCA mutation carriers to develop tumors in those organs.

3. Conclusions and final remarks

As reported at the beginning of this chapter, breast cancer is a relevant issue due to its high incidence worldwide. Here, we summarized the very first steps that resulted in the discovery of BRCA1 and BRCA2 using basic genetic and statistics tools by many groups simultaneously. Then, the prognosis of having a mutation in these genes is explained and the strategies and treatments for cancer prevention in mutant carriers are indicated. Additionally, we report the legal history around the controversial patenting of these genes as well as a brief report about Mary Claire King a key scientist in BRCA discovery and in the recent history of our country. In the second part of this chapter, we review some BRCA1 and BRCA2 biological functions, particularly those relevant to the not completely answered question of why mutations in these genes cause high risk of developing tumors particularly in hormone-responsive tissues.

In summary, it can be said that the story behind the finding of BRCA1 and BRCA2 as well as its further scientific and clinical developments have not been linear at all. It have involved multiple actors as classical and molecular geneticists, clinicians, lawyers, entrepreneurs, ethical experts, pharmaceutical companies, and the judiciary systems of diverse countries. Undoubtly, is one of the best examples of how a scientific discovery may change human society for ever.

Acknowledgements

The authors would like to thank the Argentine National Council for Scientific and Technological Research (CONICET), the University of Buenos Aires (UBA) and the National Agency for Scientific and Technological Promotion (ANPCyT) for their support.

This chapter is in memoriam of Dr. Moisés Burachik, who has always emphasized the necessity of a fluid interaction between scientific research and human society, for inspiring several generations to study and do science in Argentina.

Author details

Natalia B. Burachik[1†], Ana Laura Ortiz[2†] and Edith C. Kordon[2*]

1 INGEBI-CONICET, FCEN, University of Buenos Aires, CABA, Argentina

2 IFIBYNE-UBA-CONICET, FCEN, University of Buenos Aires, CABA, Argentina

*Address all correspondence to: ekordon@qb.fcen.uba.ar

† Equally contributed to this chapter.

References

[1] World Health Organization [Internet]. Available from: Breast Cancer. [Accessed: August 01, 2022]

[2] Winters S, Martin C, Murphy D, Shokar NK. Breast cancer epidemiology, prevention, and screening. Progress in Molecular Biology and Translational Science. 2017;**151**:1-32. p. 1-32. DOI: 10.1016/bs.pmbts.2017.07.002

[3] Hall JM, Lee MK, Newman B, et al. Linkage of early-onset familial breast cancer to chromosome 17q21. Science. 1990;**250**(4988):1684-1689. DOI: 10.1126/science.2270482

[4] Narod SA, Feunteun J, Lynch HT, et al. Familial breast-ovarian cancer locus on chromosome 17q12-q23. Lancet. 1991;**338**(8759):82-83. DOI: 10.1016/0140-6736(91)90076-2

[5] Hall JM, Friedman L, Guenther C, et al. Closing in on a breast cancer gene on chromosome 17q. American Journal of Human Genetics. 1992;**50**(6):1235-1242

[6] Miki Y, Swensen J, Shattuck-Eidens D, et al. A strong candidate for the breast and ovarian cancer susceptibility gene BRCA1. Science. 1994;**266**(5182):66-71. DOI: 10.1126/science.7545954

[7] Wooster R, Neuhausen SL, Mangion J, et al. Localization of a breast cancer susceptibility gene, BRCA2, to chromosome 13q12-13. Science. 1994;**265**(5181):2088-2090. DOI: 10.1126/science.8091231

[8] Wooster R, Bignell G, Lancaster J, et al. Identification of the breast cancer susceptibility gene BRCA2 [published correction appears in Nature 1996 Feb 22;**379**(6567):749]. Nature. 1995;**378**(6559):789-792. DOI: 10.1038/378789a0

[9] Ferla R, Calò V, Cascio S, et al. Founder mutations in BRCA1 and BRCA2 genes. Annals of Oncology. 2007;**18**(Suppl. 6):vi93-vi98. DOI: 10.1093/annonc/mdm234

[10] National Cancer Institute. BRCA Gene Mutations: Cancer Risk and Genetic Testing [Internet]. Available from: https://www.cancer.gov/about-cancer/causes-prevention/genetics/brca-fact-sheet. [Accessed: August 01, 2022]

[11] BRCA1 and BRCA2 Inherited Gene Mutations in Women [Internet]. Available from: https://www.komen.org/breast-cancer/risk-factor/topics/brca-genes/ [Accessed: August 01, 2022]

[12] Genetics of Breast and Gynecologic Cancers (PDQ®)–Health Professional Version. [Internet]. Available from: https://www.cancer.gov/types/breast/hp/breast-ovarian-genetics-pdq#_88. [Accessed: August 01, 2022]

[13] Gayther SA, Ponder BA. Mutations of the BRCA1 and BRCA2 genes and the possibilities for predictive testing. Molecular Medicine Today. 1997;**3**(4):168-174. DOI: 10.1016/S1357-4310(97)01017-4

[14] Levy-Lahad E, Lahad A, King MC. Precision medicine meets public health: population screening for BRCA1 and BRCA2. Journal of the National Cancer Institute. 2014;**107**(1): 420. Published 2014 Dec 30. DOI: 10.1093/jnci/dju420

[15] Bluman LG, Rimer BK, Berry DA, et al. Attitudes, knowledge, and risk perceptions of women with breast and/or ovarian cancer considering testing for BRCA1 and BRCA2. Journal of Clinical Oncology. 1999;**17**(3):1040-1046. DOI: 10.1200/JCO.1999.17.3.1040

[16] Jolie, Angelina. My Medical Choice. [Internet]. Available from: https://www.nytimes.com/2013/05/14/opinion/my-medical-choice.html. [Accessed: August 01, 2022]

[17] McCarthy AM, Armstrong K. The role of testing for BRCA1 and BRCA2 mutations in cancer prevention. JAMA Internal Medicine. 2014;**174**(7): 1023-1024. DOI: 10.1001/jamainternmed.2014.1322

[18] Rebbeck TR, Friebel T, Lynch HT, et al. Bilateral prophylactic mastectomy reduces breast cancer risk in BRCA1 and BRCA2 mutation carriers: the PROSE study group. Journal of Clinical Oncology. 2004;**22**(6):1055-1062. DOI: 10.1200/JCO.2004.04.188

[19] Schrag D, Kuntz KM, Garber JE, Weeks JC. Decision analysis--effects of prophylactic mastectomy and oophorectomy on life expectancy among women with BRCA1 or BRCA2 mutations [published correction appears in N Engl J Med 1997 Aug 7; 337(6): 434]. The New England Journal of Medicine. 1997;**336**(20):1465-1471. DOI: 10.1056/NEJM199705153362022

[20] Takaoka M, Miki Y. *BRCA1* gene: function and deficiency. International Journal of Clinical Oncology. 2018;**23**:36-44. DOI: 10.1007/s10147-017-1182-2

[21] Pujol P, Barberis M, Beer P, et al. Clinical practice guidelines for BRCA1 and BRCA2 genetic testing. European Journal of Cancer. 2021;**146**:30-47. DOI: 10.1016/j.ejca.2020.12.023

[22] Matthijs G. The European opposition against the BRCA gene patents. Familial Cancer. 2006;**5**(1):95-102. DOI: 10.1007/s10689-005-2580-6

[23] Lecrubier A. Patents and public health. European institutions are challenging Myriad Genetics's patent monopoly on the brca1 gene. EMBO Reports. 2002;**3**(12):1120-1122. DOI: 10.1093/embo-reports/kvf251

[24] Specter, Micheael. Can We Patent Life? [Internet]. Available from: https://www.newyorker.com/tech/annals-of-technology/can-we-patent-life. [Accessed: August 01, 2022]

[25] Williams-Jones B, Burgess MM. Democratising access to genetic services. Familial Cancer. 2006;**5**(1):117-121. DOI: 10.1007/s10689-005-2582-4

[26] Matloff E, Caplan A. Direct to confusion: lessons learned from marketing BRCA testing. The American Journal of Bioethics. 2008;**8**(6):5-8. DOI: 10.1080/15265160802248179

[27] Caulfield T, Bubela T, Murdoch CJ. Myriad and the mass media: the covering of a gene patent controversy. Genetics in Medicine. 2007;**9**(12):850-855. DOI: 10.1097/gim.0b013e31815bf965

[28] Rosenfeld JA, Mason CE. Pervasive sequence patents cover the entire human genome. Genome Medicine. 2013;**5**(3):27. Published 2013 Mar 25. DOI: 10.1186/gm431

[29] Chuang CS, Lau DT. Patenting human genes: the myriad controversy. Clinical Therapeutics. 2010;**32**(12):2054-2056. DOI: 10.1016/j.clinthera.2010.11.013

[30] Toland AE, Forman A, Couch FJ, et al. Clinical testing of BRCA1 and BRCA2: a worldwide snapshot of technological practices. NPJ Genomic Medicine;**2018, 3**(7). Published 2018 Feb 15. DOI: 10.1038/s41525-018-0046-7

[31] Sanders, Robert. Berkeley's Allan C. Wilson, The World Authority on 'Molecular Evolution,' Is Dead at 56.

[Internet]. Available from: https://www.berkeley.edu/news/media/releases/archival/allan_wilson_obit.shtml [Accessed: August 01, 2022]

[32] Neill US. A conversation with Mary-Claire King. The Journal of Clinical Investigation. 2019;**129**(1):1-3. DOI: 10.1172/JCI126050

[33] King MC. Evidence is evidence: an interview with Mary-Claire King interviewed by Jane Gitschier. PLoS Genet. 2013;**9**(9):e1003828. DOI: 10.1371/journal.pgen.1003828

[34] Rodriguez, Margarita. Cáncer de mama: Mary-Claire King, la científica que ayudó a descubrir el "gen" de la enfermedad (y el emotivo vínculo que la une a Argentina y Chile). [Internet]. Available from: https://www.bbc.com/mundo/noticias-54569982. [Accessed: August 01, 2022]

[35] UW Genome Science. Mary-Claire King. Professor of Genome Sciences and of Medicine (Medical Genetics). [Internet]. Available from: https://www.gs.washington.edu/faculty/king.htm. [Accessed: August 01, 2022]

[36] Smith S, Easton D, Evans D, et al. Allele losses in the region 17q12-21 in familial breast and ovarian cancer involve the wild–type chromosome. Nature Genetics. 1992;**2**:128-131. DOI: 10.1038/ng1092-128

[37] Hakem R, de la Pompa JL, Sirard C, et al. The tumor suppressor gene Brca1 is required for embryonic cellular proliferation in the mouse. Cell. 1996;**85**(7):1009-1023. DOI: 10.1016/s0092-8674(00)81302-1

[38] Suzuki A, de la Pompa JL, Hakem R, et al. Brca2 is required for embryonic cellular proliferation in the mouse. Genes & Development. 1997;**11**(10):1242-1252. DOI: 10.1101/gad.11.10.1242

[39] Vaughn JP, Davis PL, Jarboe MD, et al. BRCA1 expression is induced before DNA synthesis in both normal and tumor-derived breast cells. Cell Growth & Differentiation. 1996;**7**(6):711-715

[40] Scully R, Chen J, Plug A, et al. Association of BRCA1 with Rad51 in mitotic and meiotic cells. Cell. 1997;**88**(2):265-275. DOI: 10.1016/s0092-8674(00)81847-4

[41] Sharan SK, Morimatsu M, Albrecht U, et al. Embryonic lethality and radiation hypersensitivity mediated by Rad51 in mice lacking Brca2. Nature. 1997;**386**(6627):804-810. DOI: 10.1038/386804a0

[42] Zhang H, Tombline G, Weber BL. BRCA1, BRCA2, and DNA damage response: collision or collusion? Cell. 1998;**92**(4):433-436. DOI: 10.1016/s0092-8674(00)80936-8

[43] Chen J, Silver DP, Walpita D, et al. Stable interaction between the products of the BRCA1 and BRCA2 tumor suppressor genes in mitotic and meiotic cells. Molecular Cell. 1998;**2**(3):317-328. DOI: 10.1016/s1097-2765(00)80276-2

[44] Patel KJ, Yu VP, Lee H, et al. Involvement of Brca2 in DNA repair. Molecular Cell. 1998;**1**(3):347-357. DOI: 10.1016/s1097-2765(00)80035-0

[45] Chapman MS, Verma IM. Transcriptional activation by BRCA1. Nature. 1996;**382**(6593):678-679. DOI: 10.1038/382678a0

[46] Milner J, Ponder B, Hughes-Davies L, Seltmann M, Kouzarides T. Transcriptional activation functions in BRCA2. Nature. 1997;**386**(6627):772-773. DOI: 10.1038/386772a0

[47] Scully R, Anderson SF, Chao DM, et al. BRCA1 is a component of the RNA

polymerase II holoenzyme. Proceedings of the National Academy of Sciences of the United States of America. 1997;**94**(11):5605-5610. DOI: 10.1073/pnas.94.11.5605

[48] Venkitaraman AR. How do mutations affecting the breast cancer genes BRCA1 and BRCA2 cause cancer susceptibility? DNA Repair (Amst). 2019;**81**:102668. DOI: 10.1016/j.dnarep.2019.102668

[49] Liehr JG. Genotoxic effects of estrogens. Mutation Research. 1990;**238**(3):269-276. DOI: 10.1016/0165-1110(90)90018-7

[50] Shivji MKK, Renaudin X, Williams ÇH, Venkitaraman AR. BRCA2 regulates transcription elongation by RNA polymerase II to prevent R-loop accumulation. Cell Reports. 2018;**22**(4):1031-1039. DOI: 10.1016/j.celrep.2017.12.086

[51] Stork CT, Bocek M, Crossley MP, et al. Co-transcriptional R-loops are the main cause of estrogen-induced DNA damage. eLife. 2016;**5**:e17548. DOI: 10.7554/eLife.17548

Section 3

BRCA Structure and Function

Chapter 3

BRCA Biological Functions

Divya Bhargavi Pulukuri, Vijaya Babu Penke, Divya Jyothi Palati, Prudvi Raj Pulla, Shanker Kalakotla and Siddhartha Lolla

Abstract

BRCA1 and BRCA2 genes encode proteins that have important roles in DNA repair and act as tumor suppressors. Though the sequence and structure of the proteins produced by BRCA1 and BRCA2 are different, they have similar biological activities. Both BRCA gene products are reported to interact with the RAD51 protein, which is essential for DNA repair through homologous recombination. BRCA gene mutations are associated with an increased risk of solid tumors. Their ubiquitously expressed protein products are involved in essential cellular functions. The defect caused by BRCA gene mutations might be leveraged to develop new targeted cancer treatments. This chapter outlines that BRCA1 and BRCA2 have unique roles in the pathways leading to DNA double-strand break repair and clinical findings show that BRCA genes play a crucial role in a variety of biological processes.

Keywords: BRCA1, BRCA2, RAD51 protein, DNA repair, cancer

1. Introduction

Mutations in the tumor suppressor genes BRCA1 (breast cancer susceptibility gene 1) and BRCA2 have an impact on various types of cancer (breast cancer susceptibility gene 2). More than 20 years ago, researchers first discovered an association between the BRCA1 and BRCA2 genes and the risk of developing ovarian and breast cancer [1]. Stomach, prostate, pancreatic, and colorectal cancers also have been linked to genetic mutations in the BRCA gene. There is some evidence that familial ovarian and breast cancers are linked to pancreatic, stomach, and prostate cancers via mutation, which accounts for 20% of these cancers [2].

While homologous recombination mends precise DNA damage, the BRCA1 and BRCA2 proteins are vital for the process [3]. This helps to ensure that the genome retains its complete and unaltered state. Depletion of BRCA capabilities consequences in genomic instability, which further drives the oncogenic conversion of non-tumorigenic cells into tumor-initiating cells, also referred to as cancer stem cells (CSCs), and further tumorigenesis. Several investigations over the last decade have shown that cancer cells within a single tumor varied significantly in terms of their potential to initiate tumors. A CSC population is capable of long-term self-renewal and differentiation into various tumor cell types and development. In addition to the prominent genomic imbalance/instability that is connected to tumor tissues, CSCs also have a high ability to self-renew and clonogenic potential, which suggests that they may act as a catalyst for the growth of cancer [4]. consequently, intratumoral heterogeneity is contingent on the CSC's development, which is represented by the with-in quantity of newly forming tumor replicates [5].

In this chapter, we discuss the interaction between the BRCA gene and the RAD51 protein, which is important for DNA repair via homologous recombination, as well as the clinical significance and the central function of BRCA genes in a variety of biological functions.

2. BRCA genes and encoded proteins

The basic sequences of BRCA1 and BRCA2 are significantly diverse. BRCA1 (with 17q21, 17 chromosomes: 43,044,294 to 43,125,482base pairs) happens to be a 24-exon protein containing 1863 amino acids. It's made up of several domains for distinct purposes. It has the zinc-finger binding domain RING (Quite Fascinating New Gene) at the N-terminus, which is required for BRCA1 and BARD1 interaction and E3 ubiquitin ligase complex formation [6]. ABRAXAS, BRIP1/FACJ, CtIP, and 2 Phosphopeptide-binding BRCT (BRCA1 C-terminal) dominions mediate the association between BRCA1 and also its associated proteins (**Figure 1**). Exons 11–13, which encode the central region of BRCA1, are often mutated in patients with breast cancer. 2 Nuclear localization signals (NLS) along with 1 coiled-coil domain are required for the interaction of BRCA2 via PALB2 [7].

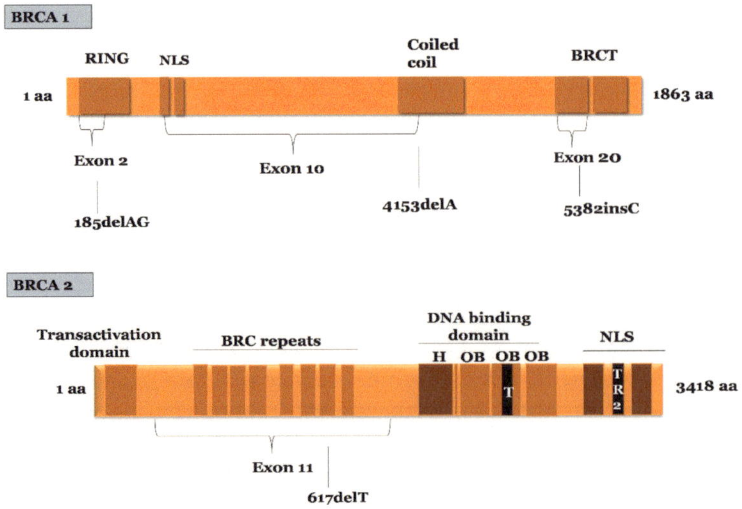

Figure 1.
Schematic representation of BRCA1 and BRCA2 proteins. BRCA1 has 23 exons and 1863 amino acids, whereas BRCA2 has 27 exons and 3418 amino acids. BRCA1 contains a highly conserved zinc-binding RING (very intriguing new gene) finger domain near the N-terminus. Two BRCT (BRCA1 C-terminal) domains are located at the C-terminus. The core region of BRCA1 is made up of two NLS (nuclear localization signals) and one coiled-coil domain. BRCA2 has eight BRC repetitions of 20–30 amino acids. BRCA2 features a TAD (transcriptional activation domain) domain at its amino-terminus and two NLS and one TR2 domain at its carboxyl-terminus. The DNA-binding domain lies at the C-terminus and consists of a helical domain (H), three oligonucleotide-binding (OB) folds, and a tower domain (T). The domain names are displayed above. Braces are used to designate exons. Below are noted the locations of founder mutations.

The BRCA1 gene has more than 1600 mutations, involving omissions, infusions, and single nucleotide mutations have been identified [8]. The majority of BRCA1 mutations have been detected in BRCT as well as RING dominions, in addition to exons from 11 to 13, that encode the NLS necessary for BRCA1 operations, then act as complex formation sites for additional BRCA1-interacting proteins, such as c-Myc, Rad50, Rad51, pRb, BRCA2 and PALB2 [9]. Ashkenazi Jews have a 5382insC frame-shift alteration that appeared in Scandinavia and Russia, as well as 185delAG founder alterations in the RING and BRCT domains [10]. Mutations in BRCA1 exons 11–13 are linked with ovarian cancer and the breast to develop pancreatic, colon, rectal, and stomach cancer [11].

BRCA2 is an enormous protein that consists of around 3418 different amino acids and is located on chromosome 13 at position 13q12.3 (base pairs 32,315,479 to 32,399,671). Its genomic data accounts for about 84.2 kb and has 27 exons. The transcriptional activation domain (TAD) is present on the N-terminus of BRCA2. Exon 11 encodes the middle region with eight RAD51-binding BRC repeats [12]. BRCA2's carboxyl terminus features a DNA-binding domain made up of a tower domain (T), 3 oligonucleotide binding (OB) folds, as well as conserved helical dominion that makes it easier for BRCA2 to attach to double- and single-stranded DNA (ssDNA) (**Figure 1**). There are 2 NLS domains and 1 TR2 domain on the C terminus of BRCA2 [13]. It has about 1800 mutations. Frameshift replacements, erasures, and nonsense genetic mutations caused by these lesions result in untimely protein curtail or non-functional proteins [14]. Exon 11 of the BRCA2 gene encodes the most common germline frameshift mutation, 6174delT. BRCA2 mutations are connected to stomach, pancreatic, breast, ovarian, prostate, gall bladder, and bile duct cancer [15].

3. Interaction of RAD51 and the BRCA proteins

Amidst changes in order and structure, BRCA1 and BRCA2 share biological roles. BRCA1 and BRCA2 have comparable subcellular localization and expression patterns. Both are expressed during the cell cycle's S phase, suggesting DNA replication responsibilities [16]. When DNA is damaged, two subnuclear foci change their distribution. Both proteins are found in synaptonemal complexes of meiotic axial filaments. This expression and localization pattern is paralleled by RAD51, a human counterpart of the bacterial protein RecA, which *E. coli* requires to repair double-strand breaks (DSBs) through genetic recombination. It's been noted that RAD51 binds to both BRCA1 and BRCA2. In vitro, BRCA2-RAD51 interacts directly with recombinant protein fragments and the yeast two-hybrid system [17]. In yeast two-hybrid tests, murine BRCA2 binding to RAD51's first 98 residues was mediated by a C-terminal motif. Human BRCA2 homologous region 95% similar to murine sequence does not bind RAD51 [18].

Eight BRC repeats mediate RAD51's interaction with human BRCA2 [19]. With the exception of BRC5 and BRC6, each repetition can bind to RAD51 independently in two-hybrid experiments and in vitro when expressed as a GST fusion protein. BRC5 and BRC6 aren't capable. In two-hybrid experiments, BRC4 binds RAD51 four times more than BRC1. PCR mutagenesis identifies a 30-residue binding consensus in BRC1 and BRC4. Despite this core motif, BRC1 and BRC4 require different residues for RAD51 binding. This shows that BRC1 and BRC4 interact differentially with RAD51 [20].

BRCA1's interaction with RAD51 was first linked to a region covering residues 758–1064 [21]. Yet it is still unknown whether direct interaction between the two proteins is possible. Co-immunoprecipitated cell extracts show a low-stoichiometry interaction not confirmed by yeast two-hybrid or recombinant proteins. In meiotic and mitotic cells, BRCA1 and BRCA2 are co-localized. A region of BRCA1 (residues 1314–1863) that is unrelated to RAD51 binding is where these two proteins interact [17]. The connection may not be direct and involves 2–5% of each protein's cellular pool. Current biochemical purification and mass spectrometry efforts to characterize the BRCA1 protein complex have not detected RAD51 or BRCA2 [22].

Therefore, of the identified physical interactions between BRCA1, BRCA2, and RAD51, the BRCA2-RAD51 contact seems to be the most well-established. Although the functional significance of their observed interactions has not yet been determined, existing data suggest that BRCA1 interacts with BRCA2, RAD51, and BRCA2 in a multimolecular complex.

4. Clinical relevance of BRCA genes

The link between BRCA1/2 domain functions and tumor growth has been studied in animal models, but clinical data are required [23]. Most BRCA gene mutations (70–80%) induce protein dysfunction or absence. Certain clinically important mutations enhance the risk of hereditary cancers [24]. In addition, numerous studies have found a correlation between BRCA1/2 mutations and aggressiveness of tumors, and inadequate clinical results in cancer patients. In a recent investigation of 603 cases of sporadic pancreatic cancer in China, it was found that the germline missense variant rs1799966 (c.4837A > G[p.Ser1613 Gly]) in the BRCT dominion of the BRCA1 gene was related to lower overall patient life expectancies [25].

Contradictory results have been found in clinical studies investigating a potential link between BRCA1 and BRCA2 mutations and the prognosis of patients with breast cancer. In a recent prospective multihospital investigation of 2733 young breast cancer patients, 388 had BRCA1/2 mutations. Overall survival did not differ between people with and without BRCA mutations. According to the analysis of 558 triple-negative breast cancer (TNBC) patients, BRCA1/2 alterations/mutation transferors outlived non-carriers overall [26]. In the same time frame, 202 invasive breast cancer patients from Japan who underwent a retrospective study discovered that a loss of heterozygosity (LOH) at the BRCA1 gene is connected to notable shorter disease-free endurance, remote metastasis-free survival, and overall endurance [27]. In yet another detailed overview, among 458 Chinese breast cancer patients with pathogenic germline BRCA2 mutations, lymph node metastases were more prevalent at diagnosis and had inferior results, such as disease-free life-span and distant relapse [28]. BRCA1 mutations enhance the prognosis for ovarian cancer, according to a meta-analysis of 33 scientific cases [29].

More prospective research on the impact of individual pathogenic mutations in tumor growth and patient responses to therapy is required to better understand how the prognosis of patients with ovarian and breast cancer is impacted by BRCA1/2 mutations. It may be possible to better target clinical treatment for BRCA-related malignancies by understanding the relationship between tumor aggressiveness and BRCA mutations.

5. Protective role of BRCA genes in the maintenance of genomic stability

Through the control of homologous recombination, the BRCA1 and BRCA2 proteins are crucial for DNA double-strand break (DSB) repair (HR) (**Figure 2**) [30]. Using a homologous template, such as sister chromatids, HR is a DNA repair technique that achieves high precision. If sister chromatids are present, they can be effective in S and G2. Pre-synapsis, post-synapsis, and synapsis are processes in DNA repair [31]. Initial DSB ends are cut during the first stage by the Mre11-RAD50-Nbs1 (MRN) complex as well as C-terminal binding protein interacting protein (CtIP) with nuclease activity, leaving a 3′- single strand (ss) DNA tail that replication protein A (RPA) protects from destruction. Next, BRCA1 and BRCA2 regulate the invasion of RAD51-ssDNA filament into homologous duplex DNA. A D-loop (displacement loop) structure is created when the third DNA strand spans between two double-stranded DNA molecules. The resulting nucleoprotein filament searches for a similar DNA sequence on the sister chromatid and enters a duplex to produce a mutual molecule. In the final stage, during post-synapsis, RAD51 separates from dsDNA. DNA polymerases stretch the damaged DNA's 3′ end, followed by DNA ligation [32]. When DNA recombination results in Holliday junctions, the various mechanisms outlined elsewhere help resolve them, leading to an error-free repair [33].

Additionally, BRCA1 controls both HR-dependent DNA repair and non-homologous end joining (NHEJ) repair. NHEJ is a DNA repair process that ligates broken DNA ends without a template. HR takes longer but is error-free and accurate at rectification. Contrarily, DNA repair by NHEJ often causes mutations. It's the fastest DNA DSB repair process. Classical (C) NHEJ occurs most often in G0 and G1 but in every phase. The process is broken down into three steps: break recognition, end-processing, and ligation. DNA-PK and NHEJ proteins are recruited when Ku70/Ku80 recognizes DSB ends. After that, DNA-PK recruits endonuclease Artemis to handle DSB ends. End ligation is promoted by the XRCC4 (X-ray repair cross-complementing protein 4)/Lig4 protein [34].

Unlike C-NHEJ, alternative (A)-NHEJ requires an MRN complex, CtIP, and poly (ADP-ribose) polymerase-1 (PARP-1) for protein recruitment and DNA lesion recognition. A-NHEJ is a backup repair route for C-NHEJ, but its mechanism is less well-known [35]. According to recent studies, dephosphorylating 53BP1 allows BRCA1 to

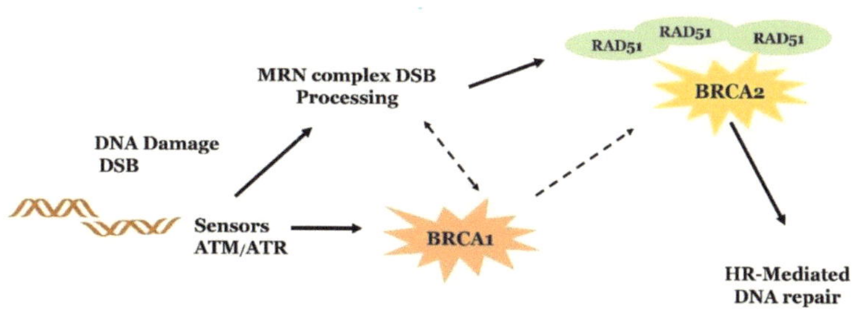

Figure 2.
The precise role of BRCA1 and BRCA2 in DNA DSB repair. The BRCA protein fixes DNA double-strand breaks, halted replication forks, and DNA cross-links. Protein kinases like ataxia telangiectasia and Rad3 related (ATR) and ataxia telangiectasia mutant (ATM) that activate the pathways are able to detect DNA damage. The RAD51 recombinase, which is responsible for mediating homology-directed (HR) repair and strand invasion is regulated by BRCA2 via the MRN complex (RAD50-MRE11-NBS1).

switch from NHEJ to HR-dependent DNA repair (p53-binding protein 1) [36]. CDK phosphorylates CtIP at Ser327 when BRCA1, CtIP, and MRN activate HR [37]. PALB2/FANCN recruits BRCA2 at DNA DSB sites during HR via BRCA1 [38].

Extensive research has also been conducted on the role of BRCA2 in DSB repair. BRCA2 plays a key function in HR by recruiting RAD51 to DSBs [39]. BRCA2 deletion causes tumorigenesis and genomic instability. This is partly because BRCA2 regulates RAD51's intracellular location and DNA-binding ability. The MRN complex recruits BRCA1 and CtIP to the DNA DSB site, which induces phosphorylation and ubiquitination. This complex promotes BRCA2 to DNA DSBs with Exo1 and DNA2-BLM (Bloom syndrome protein). BRCA2 recruits RAD51 to DNA damage sites, displacing RPA. BRCA2's BRC repeats and TR2 domain allow RAD51 to load onto ssDNA and search for a DNA template [36]. BRCA2 may work with RAD51 paralogs XRCC2 and XRCC3 to assemble RAD51 with ssDNA [38]. It regulates stalled DNA replication by binding to RAD51 BRC repeats. BRCA2 inhibits MRE11 to prevent chromosomal defects during replication stalling [40] 3′-repair exonuclease 2 (TREX-2) complexes recruit BRCA2 to handle R-loops, which form during transcription from hybrid DNA-RNA and ssDNA [41].

6. Biological functions of the BRCA gene

6.1 Role of BRCA genes in the biological response to DNA damage and DNA double-strand break repair (DSB)

BRCA1 and BRCA2 co-localize DNA damage responses were inevitable. Studies on breast-cancer-susceptibility-gene-mutated cells support this. DNA damage triggers cell cycle checkpoints and DNA repair mechanisms. Inactivating DNA checkpoints or repair enhances genotoxicity. Due to increased X-ray sensitivity, BRCA1 and BRCA2 take part in a significant role in the response to DNA damage in murine cells [42, 43]. DSB repair, the X-ray radiation-induced lesion, was found to be defective in BRCA1 or BRCA2-deficient cells. NHEJ and homologous recombination repair DSBs in mammalian cells. NHEJ ligates DNA without end-sequence homology. DSBs can be repaired by exchanging DNA from damaged templates and sister chromatids. In mammalian cells, its mechanism is unknown. Yeast recombination depends on Rad51p, Rad52p, Rad54p, Rad55p, Rad57p, Rad59p, and Mre11p/Xrs2p-Rad50. These yeast genes have similar mammalian homologs [44].

Existing research shows that BRCA2 might not be required for DSB repair through NHEJ. The V(D)J reconfiguration of T cell receptors or antibodies, known as an NHEJ reaction, can occur if the mouse Brca2 gene is shortened [42]. BRCA2-deficient cells can perform DNA-PK-dependent NHEJ in vitro [45]. BRCA2 is essential for DSB repair by homologous recombination, according to recent, convincing data. Truncated Brca2 cells develop tri-radial and quadri-radial chromosomes in culture [42]. Radial features indicate Bloom's syndrome and Fanconi's anemia. BRCA2 deficiency hinders DNA-damaged RAD51 nuclear foci and repair sites [45].

BRCA1 and BRCA2 play different roles in DSB recombination. BRCA2 appears to play a direct role in this mechanism. BRCA2 may influence RAD51's intracellular transport and function. BRCA2 may aid in the movement of RAD51 out of its synthesis site to its active position since RAD51, which lacks a nuclear localization signal, is poorly carried into the nucleus in cells with a defective form of the gene. Peptides BRC3, BRC4, or BRC7 suppress nucleoprotein filament formation in vitro. Gel filtration indicated that binding RAD51 to BRC peptides prevents filament multimerization. These data suggest that BRCA2-RAD51 cannot promote homologous recombination in vivo. These in-vitro data show that BRCA2 is necessary for DSB repair in vivo. The BRCA2-Rad51 complex may exist in two states in vivo: an inactive state that precludes Rad51 from adhering to single-strand DNA as well as an active state where Rad51 generates nucleoprotein filaments that BRCA2 can transfer. A structural change in the BRCA2-Rad51 interaction that releases Rad51 from BRCA2 may be facilitated by increased phosphorylation. This in vitro biochemical prototypical may not apply to BRCA2's cellular action. Structural analysis of BRCA2-Rad51 may shed light on this [46].

BRCA1 is also important for homologous recombination DSB repair, but its mechanism is unclear (**Figures 2** and **3**). Due to the low stoichiometry of their interaction, it might not directly affect RAD51 function. BRCA1 binds to recombination proteins besides RAD51 [22]. RAD50, MRE11, and NBS1 co-localize and coimmunoprecipitate with BRCA1, but foci localization is unknown. Recent research shows BRCA1 regulates RAD50-MRE11-NBS1. MRE11's exonuclease may repair DSBs [47]. How this process aids DNA repair is unknown. The BRCA1-complex interaction indicates proximal roles.

6.2 BRCA gene-dependent transcriptional regulation

There is evidence from numerous studies indicating the transcriptional control of genes is regulated by both the BRCA1 and BRCA2 proteins [48]. The DNA plasmid

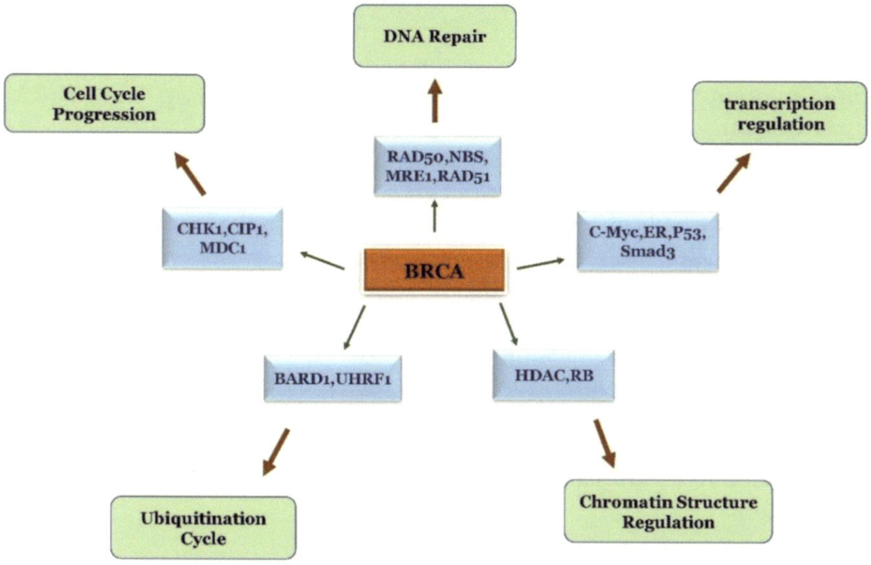

Figure 3.
Functional features of BRCA proteins. The BRCA protein has many activities in diverse biological processes including DNA repair, transcription regulation, cell cycle progression, ubiquitination cycle, and chromatin structure regulation. Proteins that are interconnecting with RAD50 double-strand break repair protein (RAD50), Nijmegen breakage syndrome (NBS), meiotic recombination homolog a (MRE1), RAD51 double-strand break repair protein (RAD51), master regulator of cellular metabolism and proliferation (C-Myc), estrogen receptor (ER), tumor protein (P53), mothers against decapentaplegic homolog 3 (Smad3), histone deacetylases (HDAC), retinoblastoma protein (RB), BRCA1 associated Ring domain 1 (BARD1), ubiquitin-like, PHD, and RING finger domain 1 (UHRF1), checkpoint kinase 1 (CHK1), cyclin-dependent kinase inhibitor 1 (CIP1), mediator of DNA damage checkpoint 1 (MDC1) in numerous cellular pathways.

that contained a BRCA1 C-terminal fragment (aa1528–1863) coupled to the yeast GAL4 (galactose–responsive transcription factor) DNA–binding dominion was used in the first investigations that revealed a role for BRCA1 in transcriptional regulation (GAL4-BRCA1). In both human and yeast cells, this recombinant protein triggered the transcription of genes. The prevalence of BRCA1 mutations in patients with breast and ovarian cancer dramatically decreased this transcriptional activity [49].

Despite the fact that the BRCA1 protein includes a DNA binding domain, recent research has shown that it is a co-regulator rather than a sequence-specific transcriptional component. Numerous transcriptional regulators, such as OCT-1, c-Myc, ER, p53, Smad3, and others, are controlled by BRCA1 [50]. For instance, BRCA1 interaction with ER controls VEGF transcription in breast cancer. It has been demonstrated that the C-terminal region of BRCA1 stimulates the p53 target gene MDM2 (Mouse Double Minute 2 Homolog) in breast cancer cells. It has been proven that BRCA1 and Smad3 work together to induce the Smad3-specific promoter. Various scientific investigations have linked BRCA2 to the control of transcription, for instance via forming a composite with p53 and Smad3 [51].

6.3 Role of BRCA gene in cell cycle progression and regulation

BRCA1 is discovered to be hyperphosphorylated in later G1 and S phases of the cell cycle and dephosphorylated in the M phase, indicating that it governs cell cycle progression, according to early research [52]. At DNA damage detectors, ATM, ATR, and Chk1 phosphorylate BRCA1 when there is DNA damage [53]. BRCA1 hinders G1/S by activating p21WAF1/CIP1. In addition to p21, the BRCA1-induced G1 arrest is dependent on Rb. BRCA1-induced G1/S arrest may be caused by the proteins ATM, ATR, BARD1, RB, p53, and p21 as well as their effectors. BRCA1-deficient cells show genomic instability, centrosome duplication, and DNA damage [54]. Also, BRCA1 acts with a DNA damage checkpoint mediator (MDC1). MDC1 recruits 53BP1, BRCA1, and MRN to DNA break spots to arrest S as well as G2/M cell cycle (**Figure 4**) [55].

The BRCA2 protein may be involved in the regulation of cell cycle progression, according to a large body of research. BRAF35/BRCA2 complexes on mitotic chromosomes phosphorylate histone H3 at Ser28 and Ser10 to aid in the condensing of mitotic chromosomes. This research verified that BRCA2/BRAF35 is crucial for cell cycle progression by microinjecting anti-BRAF35 or anti-BRCA2 antibodies into HeLa cell nuclei [56]. Recent research has shown that BRCA2-deficient cells are very susceptible to the anti-cancer medication S23906, which is attributable to both a deficiency in HR-dependent DNA repair and a malfunctioning S-phase checkpoint [57].

6.4 BRCA facilitated chromatin remodeling and regulation of epigenetic gene expression

Genome expression can be controlled by chromatin remodeling, which is regulated by BRCA1. RCA1 and its ubiquitin E3 ligase activities maintain gene silencing. Histone H2A is ubiquitinated to form heterochromatin. Tandemly repeated DNA sequences were produced when BRCA1 was deleted, a pathogenic BRCA1 mutant (T37R) was expressed, or BARD1 shRNA was used [58]. The chromatin remodeling complex SWItch/Sucrose Non-Fermentable (SWI/SNF) contains a BRG1 subunit, which BRCA1 can directly adhere to it. The dominant negative BRG1 mutant blocks p53-mediated BRCA1 transcription. BRCA1-containing chromatin remodeling complexes may lead to breast and ovarian cancer [59]. A novel BRCA1 cofactor (COBRA1)

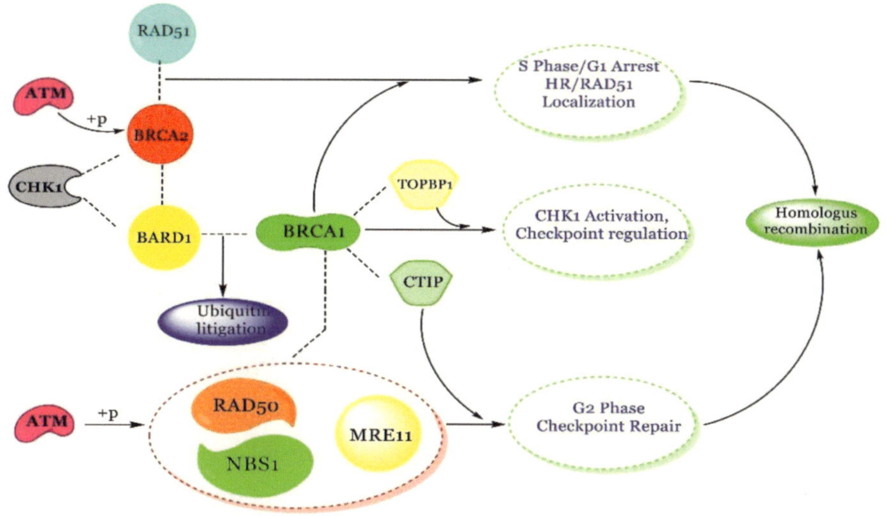

Figure 4.
The specific role of BRCA1 and BRCA2 in the regulation of the cell cycle. The proteins BRCA1 and BRCA2 and their associated proteins are responsible for cell cycle regulation. ATM and Chk1 phosphorylate BRCA1 at DNA damage detectors. BRCA1 impedes G1/S phase progression by activating TOPBP1 (topoisomerase 2- binding protein 1) and CTIP (C- terminal binding protein 1), induced G2 arrest is also dependent on RAD50 (RAD50 double-strand break repair protein), NBS1 (Nijmegen breakage syndrome 1 mutated gene), and MRE11 (meiotic recombination 11 homolog 1).

binds directly with endogenous BRCA1 and it can activate chromatin decondensation and is recruited to chromosomes by BRCA1's BRCT1 domain [60].

Oncogenic microRNAs (miR) have been linked to BRCA1 by several studies. BRCA1-HDAC2 deacetylates H2A, H3, and miR-155. BRCA1 loss and HDAC inhibitors activate MiR-155 and diminish H2A and H3 acetylation, lowering oncomiR expression [61]. High PARP breast cancers upregulate miR-151-5p. This study implies PARP drugs could target miR-151-5p in BRCA1-mutant cancer patients. BRCA1 mutations silence the PEMT gene, which produces choline, a breast tumor nutrition. The PEMT promoter −132's hypermethylation of the DNA, which raises H3K9me and lowers H3K9ac, is the mechanism underlying this epigenetic repression [62]. BRCA1 regulates sirtuin 1, a NAD-dependent histone deacetylase in cancer. Imbalanced BRCA1 and SIRT1 activity can lead to cellular transformation and tumor growth, and BRCA1 regulates transcription-silencing chromatin modification PRC2. In order for H3K27 tri-methylation, heterochromatin formation, and PRC2 occupancy on chromatin to occur, BRCA1 interacts with the oncogenic lncRNA HOTAIR [63]. These results indicate that BRCA1 inhibits PRC2 to induce breast cancer.

6.5 Degradation of the BRCA proteins via proteasomes and ubiquitination

The cell cycle regulates the post-translational activity of the BRCA1 protein. Also, tumorigenesis ubiquitinates and degrades BRCA2, causing genomic variability and non-familial cancers. Numerous proteins influence the stability of BRCA1/BRCA2, such as the cysteine protease Cathepsin S (CTSS), which binds to the BRCT dominion of BRCA1 and encourages its proteolytic destruction, the E2 ubiquitin-conjugating enzyme E2T (UBE2T), and the E3 ubiquitin ligases Herc2 and F-box protein 44. (FBXO44). BARD1 stabilizes BRCA1 expression [64].

According to Kim *et al.*, Fyn-related kinase (Frk)/Rak positively affects the stability of the BRCA1 protein by directly phosphorylating BRCA1 [61]. BRCA2 3'UTR interacts with miR-19a and miR-19b, lowering mRNA and protein levels. BRCA1/2 is regulated by protein and post-transcriptional control [65]. Chronic myeloid leukemia cells with BCR-ABL1 have less BRCA1. By attaching to 3'UTR ARE sites, the TIRA (TIA1 cytotoxic granule-associated RNA-binding protein-like1) protein prevents BRCA1 mRNA translation. HuR mRNA-binding protein improved mRNA stability and translation in the same research [66]. BRCA1 is silenced by UHRF1 (ubiquitin-like, PHD, and RING finger domain 1). By building up repressive histone marks on the promoter and restricting transcription factor binding, UHRF1 controls the transcription of BRCA1 [67].

6.6 BRCA protein function in autophagy

BRCA1 and BRCA2 are both necessary for quality control, the autophagy route for damaged mitochondria, and mitophagy. After being given oligomycin, antimycin A, or the PARP inhibitor AZD2281, mitophagy was reduced when BRCA1 and BRCA2 were knocked down. Under ER stress and serum fasting, siRNA-mediated BRCA1 knockdown induced pro-survival autophagy. BRCA1 activation triggers protective autophagy. Chemotherapeutic drugs enhanced pro-survival autophagy in BRCA1-mutated ovarian cells [68]. This study revealed that BRCA1 modulates chemotherapy-induced tumor cell death.

6.7 Classical or novel BRCA1 cytoplasmic functions

BRCA1 is widely recognized as a nucleoplasmic chromosomal caretaker. Several studies reveal BRCA1's cytoplasmic function. BRCA1 is recognized for regulating centrosomes. Centrosome amplification (CA) is common in human malignancies. CA can cause cancer and a poor prognosis [69]. BRCA1 ubiquitinates -tubulin in late S and G2/M via the BRCA1–BARD1–OLA1 complex. BRCA1 reduces early S-phase centrosome microtubule nucleation [70]. According to these results, loss of BRCA1 centrosome control may promote hypertrophy and aneuploidy in breast cancers. Cytoplasm BRCA1 is also implicated in apoptosis. BRCA1 promotes GADD45-independent apoptosis. BARD1 masks BRCA1's nuclear export signal and retains it in the nucleus. Nuclear export and cytoplasmic accumulation induce apoptosis with BRCA1 overexpression [71].

7. The consequences of the BRCA gene

When BRCA gene phenotypes are identified in malignancies, it may be possible to develop cytotoxic agent regimens that are targeted at the mechanisms that cause DNA-repair abnormalities in cancer cells. BRCA2 and other FA (Fanconi anemia) gene dysfunction cause cells to be extremely sensitive to cancer treatment that cause DNA crosslinks [72]. In contrast, Tumor cells with BRCA1 mutations are sensitive to DNA-crosslinking agents, but susceptible to mitotic-spindle poisons like taxanes [73]. Because taxanes are widely used in the treatment of breast and ovarian cancer, it's going to be essential for researchers to ascertain in clinical trials which of these tumors are resistant to taxanes. A study will randomize patients with metastatic familial-BRCA1/2 breast tumors among docetaxel and carboplatin treatment to test whether in vitro investigations translate into better clinical efficacy [74]. If employed successfully, similar techniques might be utilized to treat tumors that have the BRCA gene.

8. Concluding remarks and perspectives

The BRCA1 and BRCA2 genes encrypt proteins whose main task is to act as tumor suppressors and play a significant role in genome stability. These two genes contribute to DNA damage pathways, cell cycle, and apoptotic cascades in hereditary breast cancer. Despite changes in sequence and structure, BRCA1 and BRCA2 proteins have similar biological roles. Both BRCA gene products interact with RAD51, an important DNA-repair protein. Defective BRCA gene products impair their function as tumor suppressors, resulting in an elevated risk of cancer. An extensive study shows that BRCA1/2 gene mutations lead to the progress of breast, ovarian, and prostate cancers. BRCA-mutated malignancies are more susceptible to treatments that produce DNA DSBs, such as platinum-based drugs and PARP inhibitors. Reverting BRCA mutations that reinstate BRCA1/2 protein function is a solely clinical challenge that necessitates the careful analysis of restored gene frequencies during treatment. Notably, BRCA reversion mutations during antitumor therapy show that BRCA deficiency is crucial during oncogenesis. Combining other cancer-related therapies, CSC (cancer stem cells) therapy, and immunotherapy could resolve BRCA reversion resistance and enhance therapeutic effectiveness. Novel activities will result from the discovery of numerous additional BRCA protein binding proteins in the future. BRCA proteins' involvement in epithelial cell biology and transformation is as yet unclear.

Conflict of interest

The authors declare no conflicts of interest.

Author details

Divya Bhargavi Pulukuri[1], Vijaya Babu Penke[2], Divya Jyothi Palati[1], Prudvi Raj Pulla[3], Shanker Kalakotla[1*] and Siddhartha Lolla[4]

1 Department of Pharmacognosy, JSS College of Pharmacy, JSS Academy of Higher Education and Research, Ooty, Nilgiris, Tamil Nadu, India

2 Dr. Reddy's Institute of Life Sciences, University of Hyderabad Campus, Hyderabad, Telangana, India

3 Department of Pharmaceutical Chemistry, JSS College of Pharmacy, JSS Academy of Higher Education and Research, Ooty, Nilgiris, Tamil Nadu, India

4 Department of Pharmacology, GITAM School of Pharmacy, GITAM Deemed to be University, Hyderabad, Telangana, India

*Address all correspondence to: drshanker@jssuni.edu.in

References

[1] Miki Y, Swensen J, Shattuck-Eidens D, Futreal PA, Harshman K, Tavtigian S, et al. A strong candidate for the breast and ovarian cancer susceptibility gene BRCA1. Science. 1994;**266**(5182):66-71

[2] Cavanagh H, Rogers K. The role of BRCA1 and BRCA2 mutations in prostate, pancreatic, and stomach cancers. Hereditary Cancer in Clinical Practice. 2015;**13**(1):1-7

[3] Jiang Q, Greenberg RA. Deciphering the BRCA1 tumor suppressor network. Journal of Biological Chemistry. 2015;**290**(29):17724-17732

[4] Peitzsch C, Tyutyunnykova A, Pantel K, Dubrovska A. Cancer stem cells: The root of tumor recurrence and metastases. In: Seminars in Cancer Biology. Vol. 44. Academic Press; Jun 1 2017. pp. 10-24

[5] Kreso A, Dick JE. Evolution of the cancer stem cell model. Cell Stem Cell. 2014;**14**(3):275-291

[6] Hashizume R, Fukuda M, Maeda I, Nishikawa H, Oyake D, Yabuki Y, et al. The RING heterodimer BRCA1-BARD1 is a ubiquitin ligase inactivated by a breast cancer-derived mutation. Journal of Biological Chemistry. 2001;**276**(18):14537-14540

[7] Sy SM, Huen MS, Chen J. PALB2 is an integral component of the BRCA complex required for homologous recombination repair. Proceedings of the National Academy of Sciences. 2009;**106**(17):7155-7160

[8] Godet I, Gilkes DM. BRCA1 and BRCA2 mutations and treatment strategies for breast cancer. Integrative Cancer Science and Therapeutics. 2017;**4**(1):1-17

[9] Clark SL, Rodriguez AM, Snyder RR, Hankins GD, Boehning D. Structure-function of the tumor suppressor BRCA1. Computational and Structural Biotechnology Journal. 2012;**1**(1):e201204005

[10] Hamel N, Feng BJ, Foretova L, Stoppa-Lyonnet D, Narod SA, Imyanitov E, et al. On the origin and diffusion of BRCA1 c. 5266dupC (5382insC) in European populations. European Journal of Human Genetics. 2011;**19**(3):300-306

[11] Brose MS, Rebbeck TR, Calzone KA, Stopfer JE, Nathanson KL, Weber BL. Cancer risk estimates for BRCA1 mutation carriers identified in a risk evaluation program. Journal of the National Cancer Institute. 2002;**94**(18):1365-1372

[12] Chatterjee G, Jimenez-Sainz J, Presti T, Nguyen T, Jensen RB. Distinct binding of BRCA2 BRC repeats to RAD51 generates differential DNA damage sensitivity. Nucleic Acids Research. 2016;**44**(11):5256-5270

[13] Yang H, Li Q, Fan J, Holloman WK, Pavletich NP. The BRCA2 homologue Brh2 nucleates RAD51 filament formation at a dsDNA–ssDNA junction. Nature. 2005;**433**(7026):653-657

[14] Fackenthal JD, Olopade OI. Breast cancer risk associated with BRCA1 and BRCA2 in diverse populations. Nature Reviews Cancer. 2007;**7**(12):937-948

[15] Walsh T, Mandell JB, Norquist BM, Casadei S, Gulsuner S, Lee MK, et al. Genetic predisposition to breast cancer due to mutations other than BRCA1 and BRCA2 founder alleles among Ashkenazi Jewish women. JAMA Oncology. 2017;**3**(12):1647-1653

[16] Bertwistle D, Swift S, Marston NJ, Jackson LE, Crossland S, Crompton MR, et al. Nuclear location and cell cycle regulation of the BRCA2 protein. Cancer Research. 1997;**57**(24):5485-5488

[17] Chen J, Silver DP, Walpita D, Cantor SB, Gazdar AF, Tomlinson G, et al. Stable interaction between the products of the BRCA1 and BRCA2 tumor suppressor genes in mitotic and meiotic cells. Molecular Cell. 1998;**2**(3):317-328

[18] Aihara H, Ito Y, Kurumizaka H, Yokoyama S, Shibata T. The N-terminal domain of the human Rad51 protein binds DNA: Structure and a DNA binding surface as revealed by NMR. Journal of Molecular Biology. 1999;**290**(2):495-504

[19] Wong AK, Pero R, Ormonde PA, Tavtigian SV, Bartel PL. RAD51 interacts with the evolutionarily conserved BRC motifs in the human breast cancer susceptibility gene brca2. Journal of Biological Chemistry. 1997;**272**(51):31941-31944

[20] Chen CF, Chen PL, Zhong Q, Sharp ZD, Lee WH. Expression of BRC repeats in breast cancer cells disrupts the BRCA2-Rad51 complex and leads to radiation hypersensitivity and loss of G2/M checkpoint control. Journal of Biological Chemistry. 1999;**274**(46):32931-32935

[21] Scully R, Chen J, Plug A, Xiao Y, Weaver D, Feunteun J, et al. Association of BRCA1 with Rad51 in mitotic and meiotic cells. Cell. 1997;**88**(2):265-275

[22] Wang Y, Cortez D, Yazdi P, Neff N, Elledge SJ, Qin J. BASC, a super complex of BRCA1-associated proteins involved in the recognition and repair of aberrant DNA structures. Genes & Development. 2000;**14**(8):927-939

[23] Moynahan ME. The cancer connection: BRCA1 and BRCA2 tumor suppression in mice and humans. Oncogene. 2002;**21**(58):8994-9007

[24] Calò V, Bruno L, Paglia LL, Perez M, Margarese N, Gaudio FD, et al. The clinical significance of unknown sequence variants in BRCA genes. Cancers. 2010;**2**(3):1644-1660

[25] Zhu Y, Zhai K, Ke J, Li J, Gong Y, Yang Y, et al. BRCA1 missense polymorphisms are associated with poor prognosis of pancreatic cancer patients in a Chinese population. Oncotarget. 2017;**8**(22):36033

[26] Copson ER, Maishman TC, Tapper WJ, Cutress RI, Greville-Heygate S, AltmanDG EB, et al. Germline BRCA mutation and outcome in young-onset breast cancer (POSH): A prospective cohort study. The Lancet Oncology. 2018;**19**(2):169-180

[27] Okada S, Tokunaga E, Kitao H, Akiyoshi S, Yamashita N, Saeki H, et al. Loss of heterozygosity at BRCA1 locus is significantly associated with aggressiveness and poor prognosis in breast cancer. Annals of Surgical Oncology. 2012;**19**(5):1499-1507

[28] Wang YA, Jian JW, Hung CF, Peng HP, Yang CF, Cheng HC, et al. Germline breast cancer susceptibility gene mutations and breast cancer outcomes. BMC Cancer. 2018;**18**(1):1-3

[29] Huang YW. Association of BRCA1/2 mutations with ovarian cancer prognosis: An updated meta-analysis. Medicine. 2018;**97**(2):1-9

[30] Venkitaraman AR. Cancer suppression by the chromosome custodians, BRCA1 and BRCA2. Science. 2014;**343**(6178):1470-1475

[31] San Filippo J, Sung P, Klein H. Mechanism of eukaryotic homologous

recombination. Annual Review of Biochemistry. 2008;**77**:229-257

[32] van Gent DC, Hoeijmakers JH, Kanaar R. Chromosomal stability and the DNA double-stranded break connection. Nature Reviews Genetics. 2001;**2**(3):196-206

[33] Matos J, West SC. Holliday junction resolution: Regulation in space and time. DNA Repair. 2014;**19**:176-181

[34] Mao Z, Bozzella M, Seluanov A, Gorbunova V. Comparison of nonhomologous end joining and homologous recombination in human cells. DNA Repair. 2008;**7**(10):1765-1771

[35] Lieber MR. The mechanism of double-strand DNA break repair by the nonhomologous DNA end joining pathway. Annual Review of Biochemistry. 2010;**79**:181

[36] Fradet-Turcotte A, Sitz J, Grapton D, Orthwein A. BRCA2 functions: From DNA repair to replication fork stabilization. EndocrRelat Cancer. 2016;**23**(10):T1-T7

[37] Zhao W, Vaithiyalingam S, San Filippo J, Maranon DG, Jimenez-Sainz J, Fontenay GV, et al. Promotion of BRCA2-dependent homologous recombination by DSS1 via RPA targeting and DNA mimicry. Molecular Cell. 2015;**59**(2):176-187

[38] Orelli BJ, Bishop DK. BRCA2 and homologous recombination. Breast Cancer Research. 2001;**3**:294

[39] Yuan SS, Lee SY, Chen G, Song M, Tomlinson GE, Lee EY. BRCA2 is required for ionizing radiation-induced assembly of Rad51 complex in vivo. Cancer Research. 1999;**59**(15):3547-3551

[40] Schlacher K, Christ N, Siaud N, Egashira A, Wu H, Jasin M. Double-strand break repair-independent role for BRCA2 in blocking stalled replication fork degradation by MRE11. Cell. 2011;**145**(4):529-542

[41] Bhatia V, Barroso SI, García-Rubio ML, Tumini E, Herrera-Moyano E, Aguilera A. BRCA2 prevents R-loop accumulation and associates with TREX-2 mRNA export factor PCID2. Nature. 2014;**511**(7509):362-365

[42] Patel KJ, Veronica PC, Lee H, Corcoran A, Thistlethwaite FC, Evans MJ, et al. Involvement of Brca2 in DNA repair. Molecular Cell. 1998;**1**(3):347-357

[43] Xu X, Weaver Z, Linke SP, Li C, Gotay J, Wang XW, et al. Centrosome amplification and a defective G2–M cell cycle checkpoint induce genetic instability in BRCA1 exon 11 isoform–deficient cells. Molecular Cell. 1999;**3**(3):389-395

[44] Karran P. DNA double strand break repair in mammalian cells. Current Opinion in Genetics & Development. 2000;**10**(2):144-150

[45] Veronica PC, Koehler M, Steinlein C, Schmid M, Hanakahi LA, van Gool AJ, et al. Gross chromosomal rearrangements and genetic exchange between nonhomologous chromosomes following BRCA2 inactivation. Genes & Development. 2000;**14**(11):1400-1406

[46] Davies AA, Masson JY, McIlwraith MJ, Stasiak AZ, Stasiak A, Venkitaraman AR, et al. Role of BRCA2 in control of the RAD51 recombination and DNA repair protein. Molecular Cell. 2001;**7**(2):273-282

[47] Paull TT, Cortez D, Bowers B, Elledge SJ, Gellert M. Direct DNA binding by Brca1. Proceedings of

the National Academy of Sciences. 2001;**98**(11):6086-6091

[48] Vidarsson H, Mikaelsdottir EK, Rafnar T, Bertwistle D, Ashworth A, Eyfjord JE, et al. BRCA1 and BRCA2 bind Stat5a and suppress its transcriptional activity. FEBS Letters. 2002;**532**(1-2): 247-252

[49] Cleveland LR. Symbiosis between termites and their intestinal protozoa. Proceedings of the National Academy of Sciences. 1923;**9**(12):424-428

[50] Yi Y, Kang H, Bae I. BRCA1 and oxidative stress. Cancers. 2014;**6**(2):771-795. DOI: 10.3390/cancers6020771

[51] Preobrazhenska O, Yakymovych M, Kanamoto T, Yakymovych I, Stoika R, Heldin CH, et al. BRCA2 and Smad3 synergize in regulation of gene transcription. Oncogene. 2002;**21**(36):5660-5664

[52] Ruffner H, Verma IM. BRCA1 is a cell cycle-regulated nuclear phosphoprotein. Proceedings of the National Academy of Sciences. 1997;**94**(14):7138-7143

[53] Tibbetts RS, Cortez D, Brumbaugh KM, Scully R, Livingston D, Elledge SJ, et al. Functional interactions between BRCA1 and the checkpoint kinase ATR during genotoxic stress. Genes & Development. 2000;**14**(23):2989-3002

[54] Yarden RI, Pardo-Reoyo S, Sgagias M, Cowan KH, Brody LC. BRCA1 regulates the G2/M checkpoint by activating Chk1 kinase upon DNA damage. Nature Genetics. 2002;**30**(3):285-289

[55] Stewart GS, Wang B, Bignell CR, Taylor AM, Elledge SJ. MDC1 is a mediator of the mammalian DNA damage checkpoint. Nature. 2003;**421**(6926):961-966

[56] Marmorstein LY, Kinev AV, Chan GK, Bochar DA, Beniya H, Epstein JA, et al. A human BRCA2 complex containing a structural DNA binding component influences cell cycle progression. Cell. 2001;**104**(2):247-257

[57] Rocca CJ, Soares DG, Bouzid H, Henriques JA, Larsen AK, Escargueil AE. BRCA2 is needed for both repair and cell cycle arrest in mammalian cells exposed to S23906, an anticancer monofunctional DNA binder. Cell Cycle. 2015;**14**(13):2080-2090

[58] Zhu Q, Pao GM, Huynh AM, Suh H, Tonnu N, Nederlof PM, et al. BRCA1 tumour suppression occurs via heterochromatin-mediated silencing. Nature. 2011;**477**(7363):179-184

[59] Bochar DA, Wang L, Beniya H, Kinev A, Xue Y, Lane WS, et al. BRCA1 is associated with a human SWI/SNF-related complex: Linking chromatin remodeling to breast cancer. Cell. 2000;**102**(2):257-265

[60] Ye Q, Hu YF, Zhong H, Nye AC, Belmont AS, Li R. BRCA1-induced large-scale chromatin unfolding and allele-specific effects of cancer-predisposing mutations. The Journal of Cell Biology. 2001;**155**(6):911-922

[61] Chang S, Sharan SK. The role of epigenetic transcriptional regulation in BRCA1-mediated tumor suppression. Transcription. 2013;**4**(1):24-28

[62] Li D, Bi FF, Chen NN, Cao JM, Sun WP, Zhou YM, et al. Epigenetic repression of phosphatidylethanolamine N-methyltransferase (PEMT) in BRCA1-mutated breast cancer. Oncotarget. 2014;**5**(5):1315

[63] Wang L, Huang H. EZH2 takes the stage when BRCA1 loses. Cell Cycle. 2013;**12**(23):3575-3576

[64] Choudhury AD, Xu H, Baer R. Ubiquitination and proteasomal degradation of the BRCA1 tumor suppressor is regulated during cell cycle progression. Journal of Biological Chemistry. 2004;**279**(32):33909-33918

[65] Mogilyansky E, Clark P, Quann K, Zhou H, Londin E, Jing Y, et al. Post-transcriptional regulation of BRCA2 through interactions with miR-19a and miR-19b. Frontiers in Genetics. 2016;7:143

[66] Podszywalow-Bartnicka P, Wolczyk M, Kusio-Kobialka M, Wolanin K, Skowronek K, Nieborowska-Skorska M, et al. Downregulation of BRCA1 protein in BCR-ABL1 leukemia cells depends on stress-triggered TIAR-mediated suppression of translation. Cell Cycle. 2014;**13**(23):3727-3741

[67] Jin W, Chen L, Chen Y, Xu SG, Di GH, Yin WJ, et al. UHRF1 is associated with epigenetic silencing of BRCA1 in sporadic breast cancer. Breast Cancer Research and Treatment. 2010;**123**(2):359-373

[68] Arun B, Akar U, Gutierrez-Barrera AM, Hortobagyi GN, Ozpolat B. The PARP inhibitor AZD2281 (Olaparib) induces autophagy/mitophagy in BRCA1 and BRCA2 mutant breast cancer cells. International Journal of Oncology. 2015;**47**(1):262-268

[69] Chan JY. A clinical overview of centrosome amplification in human cancers. International Journal of Biological Sciences. 2011;7(8):1122

[70] Kais Z, Chiba N, Ishioka C, Parvin JD. Functional differences among BRCA1 missense mutations in the control of centrosome duplication. Oncogene. 2012;**31**(6):799-804

[71] Fabbro M, Schuechner S, Au WW, Henderson BR. BARD1 regulates BRCA1 apoptotic function by a mechanism involving nuclear retention. Experimental Cell Research. 2004;**298**(2):661-673

[72] Howlett NG, Taniguchi T, Olson S, Cox B, Waisfisz Q, de Die-Smulders C, et al. Biallelic inactivation of BRCA2 in Fanconi anemia. Science. 2002;**297**(5581):606-609

[73] Tassone P, Tagliaferri P, Perricelli A, Blotta S, Quaresima B, Martelli ML, et al. BRCA1 expression modulates chemosensitivity of BRCA1-defective HCC1937 human breast cancer cells. British Journal of Cancer. 2003;**88**(8):1285-1291

[74] Couzin J. Choices--and uncertainties--for women with BRCA mutations. Science. 2003 Oct 24;**302**(5645):592

Chapter 4

The Fundamental Role of BARD1 Mutations and Their Applications as a Prognostic Biomarker for Cancer Treatment

Yousef M. Hawsawi and Anwar Shams

"Our genomes carry the story of evolution, written in DNA, the language of molecular genetics, and the narrative is unmistakable."
Kenneth R. Miller
July 14, 1948

Abstract

BRCA1-associated RING domain 1 (BARD1) constitutes a heterodimeric complex with BRAC1 that triggers several essential biological functions that regulate gene transcription and DNA double-stranded break repair mechanism. BARD1 gene was discovered in 1996 to interact with BRCA1 directly and encodes a 777-aa protein. Interestingly, the BARD1 has a dual role in breast cancer development and progression. It acts as a tumor suppressor and oncogene; therefore, it is included on panels of clinical genes as a prognostic marker. Structurally, BARD1 has homologous domains to BRCA1 that aid their heterodimer interaction to inhibit the progression of different cancers, including breast and ovarian cancers. In addition to the BRCA1-independent pathway, other pathways are involved in tumor suppression, such as the TP53-dependent apoptotic signaling pathway. However, there are abundant BARD1 isoforms that are different from full-length BARD1 due to nonsense and frameshift mutations and deletions associated with susceptibility to cancer, such as neuroblastoma, lung cancer, cervical cancer, and breast cancer. In the current chapter, we shed light on the spectrum of BARD1 full-length genes and isoform mutations and their associated risk with breast cancer. The chapter also highlights the role of BARD1 as an oncogene in breast cancer patients and its uses as a prognostic biomarker for cancer susceptibility testing and treatment

Keywords: BARD1, BRAC1/BARD1, BARD1 isoforms, BARD1 mutation, breast cancer, tumor suppressor, oncogene

1. Introduction

1.1 A glance on The BRAC1/BARD1

In recent decades, cell biology and molecular genetics have revolutionized our understanding of cancer in general and breast cancer in particular. In this book, we focused on the BRCA1 and BRCA2 mutations. BRCA1-associated RING domain 1 (BARD1) is the name of a protein that Wu et al. in 1996 found as a BRCA1 (BReast CAncer type 1) binding partner [1]. Here, we shifted our focus to the BARD1 as a potential prognostic biomarker for breast cancer.

Generally, the BRAC1/BARD1 constitutes a heterodimeric complex that mediates numerous fundamental biological functions, specifically in regulating gene transcription and DNA double-stranded break repair mechanism [2, 3]. Furthermore, BRCA1 and its partner BARD1 protein are essential in other cellular processes involving chromatin remodeling, telomere regulation, replication fork maintenance, cell cycle progression, apoptosis, and tumor inhibition [4]. BRAC1/BARD1 possesses an enzymatic activity through its E3 ubiquitin ligase capacity that assists in regulating the biological processes and controlling the activity and transcription of other protein complexes [2]. BRAC1/BARD1 acts as a nucleosome reader and writer to scan and correct the DNA breaks by following the homologous recombination pathway. The C-terminal domain of BARD1 serves as a reader/scanner player, while the N-terminal domain exhibits the writer/corrector capacity. Both domains interact with a nucleosome in a wrapping fashion, activating the Ub ligase function [2]. One study has identified a negative regulator of BARD1, DCAF8L2 (a DDB1-Cullin-associated factor (DCAF) associated with CRL4 E3 ligase). The interaction between BARD1 and DCAF8L2 resulted in the degradation and ubiquitination of BARD1 with subsequent disassembly and uncoupling of the BRCA1/BARD1 complex. Additionally, DCAF8L2 expression was upregulated in breast cancer cells suggesting an oncogenic function via disrupting the BRCA1/BARD1 complex stability [3]. The BARD1 gene plays two distinct roles in cancer progression, specifically breast cancer. Thus, several biological researchers have made important discoveries about the BARD1 gene's role in cancer evolution and its potential applications as a prognostic biomarker for breast tumors, or at the very least, to consider it a possible candidate for targeted breast cancer therapy [5].

1.2 BARD1 structure, locations, and isoforms

The human BARD1 gene has 11 exons that code for a 777 aa protein with a molecular weight of 87 kDa. BARD1 was discovered in 1996 and reported to interact with BRCA1 directly through their homologous N-terminal RING domains n chromosome 2 (2q34–35) [6]. Bard1 protein is structurally made up of a RING-finger domain at the N-terminal region, three repeating Ankyrin (ANK) domains in between, and two tandems of BRCA1 domains at the C-terminal area (BRCT) [6]. Interestingly, the BRCT repeats are essential for controlling how other partners' proteins interact with one another in a phosphorylation-based manner. These interactor proteins are crucial to mediate crucial cellular processes, including DNA damage checkpoints, DNA repair machinery, and cell cycle regulation [7, 8]. Notably, the RING-finger domain and BRCT repeats are essential for the BRCA1-BARD1 complex's ability to suppress cancer [9, 10]. The presence of several exomes in full-length BARD1 (FL-BARD1, resulted in different isoforms) **Figure 1** represents a scaled diagram depicting the comparison of protein structures of BARD1, BRCA1, and BRCA2

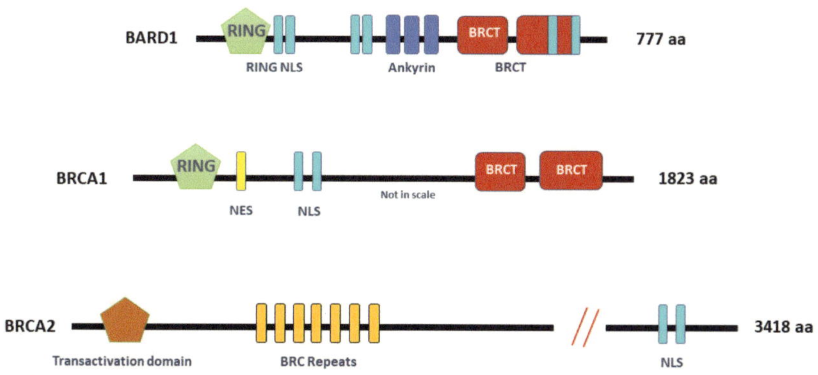

Figure 1.
A scaled diagram depicting the comparison of protein structures of BARD1, BRCA1, and BRCA2. The diagram illustrates the different protein structures of BARD1, BRCA1, and BRCA2. BRCT (dark red), RING (green), and ankyrin (dark blue) domains. The putative nuclear localization signals (NLS, light blue) and the nuclear export signal (NES, yellow) are shown. The location of BARD1's third NLS, at amino acid residue 321, is crucial for nuclear localization. With eight copies of a 70 amino acid motif known as the BRC repeats and a conserved transactivation domain (TD), BRCA2 is entirely unrelated to either BARD1 or BRCA1.

There are many BARD1 isoforms with skipped exons and various molecular weights [11]. The isoforms are more frequently found in association with cancerous cells [12, 13]. For instance, isoform α has skipped exon 2. While the isoform β skipped exons 2 and 3, which causes the open reading frame (ORF) to a frameshift, resulting in the translation of shorter proteins (758 aa (85 kDa) and 680 aa (75 kDa), respectively. However, isoform γ is typically interrupted by the deletion of exon 4. Isoforms φ and δ skipped exons 2–6 and 3–6 to produce 326aa (37 kDa) and 307 aa (35 kDa) proteins, respectively. Isoform ε skipped exons 4–9, resulting in a protein with a molecular weight of 30 kDa (264 aa), while the skipping of exons 1, 10, and 11 leads to isoform η. Another splicing from exons 1 to 10 is worthwhile since it interrupts the ORF. As a result, additional alternative ORFs may host the translation's start codon,

No.	BARD1 isoform	Amino acid	Molecular weights	Corresponding exons skipping	Associated cancer phenotypes
1	isoform α	758 aa	85 kDa	lacks exon 2	
2	β isoform	680 aa	75 kDa	lacks exons 2 and 3	
3	isoform γ			exon four deletion	
4	isoforms φ	326aa	37 kDa	missing exons 2–6	HeLa and ovarian cancer cells
5	isoforms δ	307 aa	35 kDa	missing exons 3–6	HeLa and ovarian cancer cells
6	isoform ε	264 aa	30 kDa	lack of exons 4–9	
7	isoform η	167 aa	19 kDa	lack of exons 1, 10, and 11	

Table 1.
Summarizes the different BARD1 isoforms.

producing a short protein with 167 amino acids (19 kDa). Surprisingly, most of these isoforms had agonistic cancer susceptibility potential because they lack the RING finger and ankyrin repeats, which are essential for the full-length BARD1's tumor suppressor capabilities [14, 15]. **Table 1** summarizes the different BARD1 isoforms.

Since we highlighted some important aspects of the BARD1 structure, it is worth highlighting the function of the Bard1 protein.

1.3 BARD1 as a tumor-suppressor gene and oncogene

The Bard1 protein performs a tumor suppressor function in BRCA1-dependent and -independent pathways. Due to their homologous domains, the BRCA1/BARD1 heterodimer can be configured by the N-terminal RING-finger domains, altering the ubiquitin ligase's activity, which controls the cell cycle chromatin structure and hormone signaling pathways as well as DNA damage response pathways [16, 17]. BRCA1-BARD1 heterodimers are disrupted by mutations in cancer cells, which results in the degradation of both proteins [1].

Technology advancements have made it clear that numerous genes, including BRCA1/2 and BARD1, play a crucial role in hereditary and familial breast cancer and ovarian cancer [18, 19]. Research has identified BARD1's function in the BRCA1-dependent pathway as an anti-breast cancer agent [20]. Because it activates ubiquitination through E3 ubiquitin ligase activity and starts the degradation process for the damaged proteins, the BARD1-BRCA1 complex is essential to the DNA damage machinery [16]. The involvement of BARD1 and BRCA1 in a homology-directed repair (HDR) of chromosomal breaks that clarifies their presence alongside RAD51 in response to DNA damage was previously discussed by Westermark et al. [21–23]. Furthermore, through a particular interaction with the poly (ADP-ribose), the BARD1 BRCT domain promotes the early recruitment of the BRCA1/BARD1 heterodimer to DNA damage sites (PAR) [24]. Studies have also demonstrated that disruptive mutations in the phosphate-binding pocket of the BARD1 BRCT domain in mice (S563F and K607A) hinder the recruitment of the BRCA1/BARD1 heterodimer to the stalled replication fork (SRF), which ultimately causes chromosomal instability [25]. Such mutations do not affect recruitment to HDR [25], contrasting with the comparable modification in BRCA1 BRCT (S1598F) [10]. Additionally, BARD1 or BRACA1 mutations linked to the prevalence of breast cancer, such as alterations in the RING finger domain, interfered with the BRCA1/BARD1 heterodimer interaction [26, 27], missense mutations [28–30], and ANK sequences that are involved in the regulation of transcription [31]. Additionally, the heterodimer prevents inappropriate mRNA polyadenylation at DNA repair sites with cleavage stimulation factor subunit 1 (CSTF1) [32, 33]. Through the ubiquitination pathway, BRCA1/BARD1 also aids in the prevention of tumor growth [34] and BRCA1's subcellular location [35].

BARD1 also acts as a tumor suppressor in a BRCA1-independent manner by interacting with the repetitive regions of the BCL3 ankyrin domains and altering the transcription factor activities of NFKB in the TP53-dependent apoptotic signaling pathway [36, 37]. Furthermore, a decrease in Bard1 expression has been linked to cellular changes related to a premalignant phenotype [38]. BARD1 has a role in preserving genomic integrity, and BRCA1 null animals were also discovered to have this trait. Early embryonic death was caused by chromosomal instability and BARD1 damage or total deletion [39]. RNA polymerase II was shown to be ubiquitinated by BARD1, and its transcription of damaged DNA was inhibited [34], ubiquitination, beta, and other processes crucial to breast cancer growth [40]. Together, these actions help FL-BARD1 to play a tumor suppressor role, in contrast to reports that BARD1 isoforms such as BARD1 work against this function and accelerate cancer development [41].

More recently, the Exome Sequencing Project and Exome Aggregation Consortium used 1915 patients to link the BARD1 gene and ovarian cancer [42], where the BARD1 gene has a mutation frequency of 0.2%. BARD1 is currently being studied to be included in panels of clinical gene testing for cancer susceptibility due to compelling data linking BARD1 mutations and breast/ovarian cancer susceptibility [43]. Since we mentioned the function of the BARD1 gene as a tumor suppressor, now we should turn to the other vital function of some isoforms of the BARD1 gene as an oncogene.

BARD1 has about 19 distinct expressed isoforms that have been identified so far [12, 44]; several of these isoforms, including BARD1β, BARD1κ, and BARD1π, have been implicated in the development of cancer by an oncogenic role [12, 13]. At the same time, it has been noted that the FL- BARD1, either on its own or in combination with BRCA1, has a tumor suppressor function [41]. However, BARD1β and BARD1δ were previously reported to have an antagonistic effect on full-length BARD1, resulting in oncogenicity and cancer susceptibility [12]. The majority of BARD1 isoforms possess BRCT domains but lack the RING finger domain necessary for the formation of BRCA1 heterodimers. Non-small cell lung cancer (NSCLC), colon cancer, breast cancer, and ovarian cancer all have abnormal BARD1 isoforms, which play a part in cancer progression and carcinogenesis. Additionally, it was revealed that the expression of BARD1 isoforms is significantly linked to a decline in the survival rate of patients with malignancies [12, 15].

BARD1 isoform anomalies result from protein translation from a different open reading frame (ORF). For instance, BARD1 can be translated as a noncontinuous ORF beginning with exon three and then exons 4 through 11. Additionally, it has been demonstrated that BARD1 isoforms inhibit the BRCA1-BARD1 ubiquitin ligase activity necessary to cause the death of cancer cells [12, 15, 40]. Furthermore, the expression of BARD1β has been associated with impaired homologous recombination (HR) and negatively impacted ubiquitin ligase activity in PARPi-sensitive colon cancer cells [45]. The epigenetic has a profound role in BARD1 gene expression and biological consequences. So, the question now is what is this role?

1.4 The epigenetic effect on BARD1 gene expression and biological consequences

Exons 6 to 11 (truncated isoforms) of the BARD1 gene were strongly expressed in Acute myeloid leukemia (AML) in vivo blasts compared to the BARD1-FL expression level. Lepore et al. demonstrated that HDACi (Vorinostat) treatment epigenetically controls the expression of BARD1 mRNA in AML cells, MCF-7 breast cancer cell line, and Kelly neuroblastoma cells. An increase in miR-19a and miR-19b levels were observed after vorinostat therapy, and when BARD1 3'UTR expression was targeted, this increased the apoptotic activity of malignant breast cells [46]. Following a similar pattern, estrogen also activated the estrogen response element (ERE) on BARD1's intron 9, which favorably controlled the protein expression of BARD1 [47].

While BARD1 9'L, a particular mutation of the BARD1 gene, was reported to compete with miRNAs (such as miR-101 and miR-203) on their binding sites of BARD1 3'UTR, it was also identified to act as competing for endogenous RNA (ceRNA) that negatively controls the expression of BARD1 mRNA [16]. The long non-coding RNAs (lncRNAs) display gene regulatory roles that modulate different biological mechanisms. GUARDIAN, a p53-responsive lncRNA, was determined to be involved efficiently in preserving genomic integrity and delivering protection against genotoxic stress. Additionally, GUARDIAN can facilitate the heterodimerization of BRCA1 with its partner interactor, BARD1, by acting as an RNA scaffold. Therefore, the breakdown of the BRCA1-BARD1 complex caused by GUARDIAN suppression increased the adverse effects of genotoxic stress, induced apoptosis, and caused genomic instability [48].

BRCA1 and BARD1 significantly influence the ATM/ATR pathway for DNA repair mechanisms important for a cell's decision to die. The BARD1 gene's epigenetic regulation was affected by histone modification of hESC. Splicing process regulation by H3K36 decreased BARD1 expression, suppressing the ATM/ATR signaling pathways that control hESC development [49]. Hepatocellular carcinoma (HCC) patients whose livers had developed cirrhosis were studied, and it was discovered that the BARD1 gene had much lower levels of methylation (13.3 percent) than in healthy controls. Additionally, it was proposed that BARD1 hypomethylation could be a biomarker for predicting aggressive illness in patients who do not have HBV [50]. Before we address the association of the BARD1 variant to breast cancer risk, we should have a breast cancer mutation in general.

1.5 Breast cancer mutations

The multiple risk factors that have been linked to the development of breast cancer include both genetic and environmental elements. To comprehend the pathogenesis and create a treatment plan, it is essential to identify the genetic and hereditary factors [51]. Numerous genes, including PALB2, ATM, BARD1, BRCA1, BRCA2, and CHEK2, have significantly maintained DNA fidelity and genomic integrity [52–54]. They are also essential in controlling the HR mechanics. As a result, it has been discovered that various mutations in genes are linked to an increased risk of developing many hereditary malignancies [55], including breast, prostate [56], ovarian, and pancreatic cancers [56–59]. Several vital polymorphisms in the domains of the BRCA1/BARD1 protein-protein interaction (PPI) complex, including M18K, V11G, L22S, and T97R, were identified by a thorough mutational investigation. These mutations also impacted the stability of the BRCA1/BARD1 PPI complex [60]. The development of preventive and therapeutic strategies to thwart the advancement of breast cancer can therefore be facilitated by a thorough understanding and investigation of the interplay between the BRCA1 and BARD1 platforms [4].

A patient with a breast cancer diagnosis and a family history of the disease was seen as a significant factor in the hereditary predisposition to the condition. BRCA1, BRCA2, PTEN, TP53, CDH1, and STK11 are rare but highly penetrant genes that account for about 30% of hereditary breast cancer cases. BRCA1 mutations were initially found in families with a similar pedigree in 1990. The BRCA2 gene variations were discovered four years later [61]. Hereditary Breast/Ovarian Cancer (HBOC) syndrome is caused by BRCA1 or BRCA2 mutations, yet some with this syndrome were negative for BRCA1 and BRCA2 mutations. BRCA1/2-mutant tumors have a basal, extremely aggressive character. Additionally, 2%–3% of breast cancer cases were found to have mutations in the uncommon but moderately penetrance genes, including; CHEK2, PALB2, ATM, RAD50, BRIP1, RAD51C, NBN, and MRE11. These genes engaged in DNA repair processes and interacted with BRCA1/2. A small number of SNPs, including the mutations for RAD51D, BARD1, RAD51C, ABRAXAS, NBN, and XRCC2BRIP, were linked to poor penetrance alleles and an increase in the risk of breast cancer in a polygenic manner. Clinical testing for mutations found in the high penetrance gene set was typically done on individuals with suspected genetic risk [62]. In addition, a genome-wide association study (GWAS) of breast cancer reported the discovery of 65 novel loci, including FES, MAP3K11, CLK2, GRK7, USP25, DFFA, PKP1, and ZKSCAN3, that are notably related with a high risk of breast cancer at $P < 5 \times 10^{-8}$ [63].

1.6 The significance of BARD1 in genetic predisposition to breast cancer

Many comprehensive sequencing studies have discovered several genetic variations among different clinical samples. Whereas the biological roles of BRCA1 have been exceptionally well documented, the functional machinery of BARD1 hasn't been fully understood. Two BARD1 cis mutations, P24S and R378S, were identified in a hereditary breast and ovarian malignancies report. BARD1 and BRCA1interaction m's affinity is decreased by the P24S mutation, whereas the R378S variant prevents the BRCA1/BARD2 complex from moving into the nucleus. The simultaneous presence of these two mutations contributed synergistically to tumor progress in vitro and in vivo models. Additionally, these two mutations mutually impair the DNA damage response, imposing genomic stability, although neither mutation alone can have a harmful effect [64]. Seven polymorphisms, including somatic missense mutations and germline modifications, were identified within the coding sequence of BARD1 in mutational research that included a variety of gynecological malignancies, ovarian, breast, and uterine tumors. These mutations caused the loss of the wild-type BARD1 allele, which led to the growth and spread of malignancies. A woman with breast and endometrial cancer presented simultaneously had the BARD1 mutation (Gln564His) [65]. Furthermore, the Gln564His mutation of BARD1 was reported to avoid p53-dependent apoptosis by reducing binding to the polyadenylation cleavage specification complex (CSTF-50) [33, 36].

Three non-synonymous variants in the BARD1 gene (Pro24Ser, Arg378Ser, and Val507Met) were assessed in a case-control analysis of 507 Chinese women with breast cancer and 539 matched controls. These SNPs demonstrated significant reductions in breast cancer risk and limited penetrance effects in the BARD1 gene on breast cancer propensity [66]. On the other hand, a large case-control study was carried out among the European (Polish and Belarusian) population to investigate the impact of the nonsense mutation c.1690C>T (p.Q564X). This nonsense variant was found to have a low/moderate increase in breast cancer risk (OR = 2.30, p = 0.04). The risk was further elevated in breast cancer forms that are more aggressive; TNBCs, bilateral breast cancers, early-onset cancer, and hereditary breast and ovarian cancers are a few examples [67]. According to the European study, the BARD1 mutation, one of the most prevalent non-BRCA1/2 mutations, was identified in 10901 TNBC cases and demonstrated a significant contribution to TNBC propensity with an incidence of 0.5–0.7%. Furthermore, Caucasian PVs American carriers of BARD1 gene pathological variants were at lower risk of TNBC (21%) than African American carriers of BARD1 gene mutations (39%) [41, 68].

To categorize the exon mutation of the BARD1 gene in 60 early-onset breast cancer patients and 240 healthy controls, direct sequencing and SNaPshot analysis were used. BARD1's rs28997575 site was found to have a deletion mutation, which increased the incidence of breast cancer by 3.4 times (P = 0.013) compared to the unaffected group. On the other hand, it was discovered that a different GC genotype missense mutation at the rs2229571 location of BRDA1 was associated with a 72.6 percent (P = 0.001) decreased risk of breast cancer. Remarkably, compared to the control group, the majority of variant carriers have a long family history of breast cancer. Highlighting the significant contribution of breast cancer-positive family history to the elevated risk of breast cancer due to genetic predisposition, especially in BARD1 polymorphism carriers [69]. Likewise, several pathogenic variants (PVs) of the BARD1 gene were compiled in a sizable pooled analytical research of both breast cancer (48,000 cases) and ovarian cancer (20,800 cases). These BARD1 PVs had a moderate chance of developing breast cancer (odds ratio (OR) = 2.90, 95 percent confidence intervals [CIs]: 2.25–3.75, p 0.0001) but not ovarian cancer (OR = 1.36, CIs: 0.87 to 2.11, p = 0.1733). As a result, the BARD1 gene has been suggested as a diagnostic biomarker for evaluating breast cancer patients [70].

More recently, three BARD1 inherited missense mutations were found in the RING domain (Cys53Trp, Cys71Tyr, and Cys83Arg) in a family diagnosed with breast malignancy. However, according to the study, the mutant BARD1/BRCA1 complex was unable resulting nucleosomes and resulted in a loss of H2A ubiquitylation. Mutant BARD1 could heterodimerize with BRCA1 due to its mutations. These mutations also activate a defect in transcriptional repression of the BRCA1-regulated estrogen metabolism genes CYP1A1 and CYP3A4, which are usually controlled by the H2A ubiquitylation pathway [71]. 76 BARD1 cancer-associated missense and truncation variants were effectively identified in a whole-exome sequencing analysis on 10,000 cancer samples from 33 cancer types. Significantly, just two known benign mutations were found to be connected to HDR, whereas four pathogenic mutations are not linked to HDR. DNA damaging agents were more sensitive to BARD1 mutant cells [72]. BARD1 is believed to be a gene predisposing to triple-negative breast cancer and a breast cancer susceptibility gene [68]. With an incidence of 0.5–0.7%, BARD1 was statistically substantially related to a moderate to high risk of TNBC. A rare missense mutation of BARD1 gene c.403G>A or p.Asp135Asn was noticed in TNBC patients. This mutation was reported to increase the response of breast cancer cells to PARPi therapy [73]. While additional BARD1 isoforms are highly expressed in several types of cancer, their common pathogenic effect is owing to the expression of the oncogenic dominant-negative form and alternative splicing (**Table 2**) [15, 74].

BARD1 gene polymorphism was found in cases of neuroblastoma and breast cancer cases. The probability of developing neuroblastoma was strongly correlated with three BARD1 gene polymorphisms (rs7585356 GNA, rs6435862 TNG, and rs3768716 ANG). Using the TaqMan approach on 145 cases and 531 controls, only the rs7585356 GNA polymorphism demonstrated notable findings in relation to higher vulnerability to nephroblastoma (odds ratio (OR) = 1.78, 95 percent confidence interval (CI) = 1.01–3.12) with stage I + II clinically [76]. The impact of eleven BARD1 SNPs on NB development has been studied in a Chinese publication. Seven out of eleven BARD1 SNPs revealed an increased risk of high stage (III/IV) NB occurrence. One SNP in the 5'-UTR (rs17489363 G > A), two SNPs in exon (rs2229571 G > C and rs3738888 C > T), and four SNPs in intron (rs3768716 A > G, rs6435862 T > G, rs3768707 C > T, and rs17487792 C > T), were among the eleven BARD1 SNPs [77]. According to reports, the variant (rs17489363 G > A) in the BARD1 gene, which is tied to NB and linked to a decrease in BARD1-FL transcription, is the most common SNP in the gene [50].

Exon 5 is frequently skipped due to the mutation c.1361C>T, which interferes with ANK repeat domains, a critical component of the splicing factor SC35 that regulates apoptosis in the ovarian cancer cell line. NuTu-19 [78]. The NuTu-19 cell line was resistant to the induction of apoptosis. Still, after exogenous expression of the entire gene BARD1, it became susceptible to apoptosis, indicating that the absence of exon 5 results in abnormal isoforms that have lost their capacity to suppress tumors and affect the apoptosis pathway [79]. The BARD1 mutations c.1977A > G, p.Gln715Ter,

No.	Exon	Nt change	Effect on protein	Frequency for heterozygotes	Previously reported in reference
1	4	1126G → C	Thr351Thr	17.3% (9/52)	[28, 75]
2	4	1145del21	7 aa deletion	1.9% (1/52)	[28, 30]
3	4	1207G → C	Arg378Ser	40.4% (21/52)	[29, 75]
4	6	1591C → T	His506His	7.7% (4/52)	[30, 75]
5	6	1592G → A	Val507Met	50% (26/52)	[28, 30, 75]
6	7	1743G → C	Cys557Ser	1.9% (1/52)	[28, 75]
7	10	2045C → T	Arg658Cys	1.9% (1/52)	[28, 75]

Table 2.
BARD1 variants in breast cancer predisposition.

c.2148delCA, and p.Thr716fs*12 have also been associated with other gynecological cancers, including fallopian tube, ovarian, and cervical cancers [79–81].

These findings from mounting data have collectively led to the conclusion that there is a context-dependent high/moderate risk of breast cancer associated with specific BARD1 SNPs. Therefore, additional practical and experimental studies are required to validate the aforementioned facts further.

1.7 Correlation between The Cys557Ser BARD1 mutation and risk of breast cancer

One meaningful known change to BARD1 is a missense mutation that causes the amino acid cysteine to be swapped out for the amino acid serine at position 557 (Cys557Ser) [75]. The 126 Finnish breast and ovarian cancer cases were used in a mutational analysis study to examine the possible impact of BARD1 alterations on tumor formation. Breast cancer cases were more likely to have the Cys557Ser missense mutation than healthy controls (7.4 vs. 1.4 percent, p = 0.001). To alter the transcriptional and apoptotic machinery, this variation is required. Intriguingly, the index cases were negative for BRCA1 and BRCA2 mutations highlighting that the occurrence of this mutation in familial predisposition to breast cancer is sufficient to cause the disease on its own [75]. In a study after this one, Stacey et al. and his colleague investigated the relationship between BARD1 Cys557Ser mutation and a familial group of breast cancer using a dataset of 1,090 Icelandic breast cancer patients with invasive type and 703 controls. Carriers of this variant are more likely than non-carriers to develop lobular and medullary breast carcinomas as single or multiple primary breast cancers. Additionally, this risk increased to 0.047 among individuals with the BARD1 Cys557Ser mutation and the BRCA2 999del5 mutation (OR 14 3.11, 95 percent CI 1.16–8.40, p 14 0.046) [82]. A case-control study of the Spanish and South American populations supported past investigations. Despite having a strong family history of breast cancer, the selected individuals have intact BRCA1/2 genes with no mutations. Examining the C-terminal of BARD1 Cys557Ser revealed a substantial increase in the risk of breast cancer (P = 0.04, OR = 3.4 [95 percent CI 1.2–10.2]). This likelihood was further elevated in patients with a family history of breast and ovarian cancer who were also found to have the BARD1 Cys557Ser joint mutation and the XRCC3 241Met variant (P = 0.02, OR = 5.01 [95 percent CI 1.36–18.5]) among patients with a family history of breast and ovarian cancer [83].

Contrarily, a study of Australian patients with a family history of breast cancer revealed that the frequency of the BARD1 Cys557Ser variant was not substantially different from case-control cases (P0.3) and was not linked to an increased risk of breast cancer [84]. Similar to the Australian findings, numerous additional studies have been unable to establish a direct connection between the BADR1 variation and the development of breast cancer [85–87]. In a cohort of 5,546 BRCA1 and 2,865 BRCA2 mutation carriers, the function of the BARD1 Cys557Ser variation or BARD1 haplotypes as modifiers of BRCA1/2 linked with breast cancer risk was further evaluated. In both BRCA1 and BRCA2 mutation carriers, with a combined expected effect of 0.90 and 0.87, respectively, there was no evidence of either BARD1 mutation to indicate a significant connection with breast cancer risk [88]. Another team of researchers employed DHPLC analysis to identify nine BARD1 coding mutations, including two novel variants, in 210 breast cancer families of Australian descent (129 of which do not have BRCA1 or BRCA2 mutations) (Thr598Ile and Ile692Thr). Yet none of these mutations harbor a pathogenic impact based on their segregation, distribution, and frequency among the selected cases. In addition, non-pathogenic polymorphisms were found in the three variants (1139del21, G1756C, and A2285G) connected to breast cancer in other populations. Therefore, it was not advised in the Australian population to use BARD1 mutations or polymorphisms as a high penetrance susceptibility gene in the progression of familial breast cancer [87].

Collectively, studies linking this BARD1 Cys557Ser mutation to breast cancer incidence have been conducted in Iceland, Finland, Spain/South America, and Italy; however, other studies involving Yoruba, Chinese, Japanese, Australians, and African-Americans have shown different results [30, 65]. These contradictory results regarding the BARD1 Cys557Ser variant's relationship to familial breast cancer susceptibility raise the possibility that this mutation is restricted to a particular geographic substructure of the European population (as a result of regional migration) rather than being a de novo variant [82]. There are several reported BARD1 mutations, and it is worthwhile to highlight their impact on cancer predisposition risk.

1.8 BARD1 gene as a potential target of new anticancer therapies including sensitivity to chemotherapy with a focus on breast cancer

BARD1 has the potential to be a new target for the therapy of breast cancer, according to several research. According to Zhu Y et al. [14], tamoxifen-resistant breast cancer cells exhibit considerably greater BARD1 and BRCA1 expression levels, which confers resistance to treatment that causes DNA damage such as cisplatin and Adriamycin but not paclitaxel [89–92]. Watanabe et al. used bisulfite-pyrosequencing to study the aberrant DNA methylation status of the BARD1 gene in 30 TNBC core biopsy specimens from patients with pathologic complete response (noninvasive cancer) and noncomplete response after neoadjuvant chemotherapy (NACT). Even though BRCA1 gene hypermethylation is linked to the TNBC subtype and may affect chemosensitivity and progression under NACT, BARD1 gene hypermethylation only showed a low-to-moderate impact on these procedures [93]. Contrarily, the González-Rivera and his colleagues 2016 underline the low incidence and uncertain clinical implications of gene mutations other than BRCA1/2 (including BARD1) and the associated unfavorable outcomes for patients with breast cancer undergoing NACT [94]. Yet more recent research revealed that tamoxifen-resistant breast cancer cells had increased BRCA1 and its related protein BARD1, making them resistant to treatment that damages DNA [95]. Neoadjuvant chemotherapy now contributes significantly to breast cancer chemotherapy and is a transitional step to adjuvant regimens and other treatments [96]. It is crucial and beneficial to increase research into BARD1's role in chemotherapy in women who are scheduled for NACT. Both ovarian and breast cancer patients with BRCA1 mutations who initially responded to platinum and PARPi therapy eventually developed resistance to both drugs [97]. In some populations, especially those with evidence of a higher occurrence of BARD1 gene mutations, it is fair to test BARD1 gene isoforms. Additionally, this method would need to be studied for its applicability to outcomes, survival rates, quality of life, influence on treatment choices, and cost-effectiveness for all patients with breast cancer.

2. Concluding remarks and perspectives

This chapter looks at the BRAC1/BARD1, a heterodimeric complex that mediates several biological functions regulating gene transcription and DNA double-stranded break repair mechanism. Then the authors moved to address the BARD1 gene structure, locations, and different isoforms. The authors also focused on the dual function of the BARD1 gene as a tumor-suppressor gene and oncogene. The authors highlighted the epigenetic effect on BARD1 gene expression and biological consequences before turning into breast cancer mutations. We emphasize the significance of BARD1 in genetic predisposition to breast cancer. We also focused on the correlation between the Cys557Ser BARD1 mutation and the risk of breast cancer. Finally, we addressed the BARD1 gene as a potential target of new anticancer therapies, including sensitivity to chemotherapy focused on breast cancer. According to our analysis of the BARD1 gene's structure and activities, this gene may be crucial to the pathogenesis of breast cancer and the mechanisms underlying cancer cells' chemo-resistance. In some populations, especially those with evidence of a higher occurrence of BARD1 gene mutations, it is fair to test BARD1 gene isoforms. Additionally, this method would need to be studied for its applicability to outcomes, survival rates, quality of life, influence on treatment choices, and cost-effectiveness for all patients with breast cancer, despite the fact that data on individuals undergoing NACT for breast cancer who have BARD1 gene polymorphism are scarce. Nevertheless, changes in gene expression following NACT may provide insight into the pathophysiology of this complex disease. Regardless of technological advances, there are still some future challenges in including the BARD1 in routine screening—theses challenges including the cost, the technologies sensitivities, and diversity of populations. More work is needed to discover more isoforms for the BARD1. However, limitations are currently present in employing a BARD1 mutation detection panel for breast cancer, such as the lacunae or lack of strong correlation of BARD1 polymorphisms in genetic predisposition to various types of cancer.

Acknowledgements

The King Faisal Specialist Hospital and Research Center in Jeddah and Taif University are gratefully acknowledged by the authors for their help and support.

Author details

Yousef M. Hawsawi[1,2*] and Anwar Shams[3]

1 King Faisal Specialist Hospital and Research Center, Jeddah, Saudi Arabia

2 College of Medicine, Al-Faisal University, Riyadh, Saudi Arabia

3 Department of Pharmacology, College of Medicine, Taif University, Taif, Saudi Arabia

*Address all correspondence to: hyousef@kfshrc.edu.sa

References

[1] Wu LC, Wang ZW, Tsan JT, Spillman MA, Phung A, Xu XL, et al. Identification of a RING protein that can interact in vivo with the BRCA1 gene product. Nature Genetics. 1996;**14**(4):430-440

[2] Witus SR, Zhao W, Brzovic PS, Klevit RE. BRCA1/BARD1 is a nucleosome reader and writer. Trends in Biochemical Sciences. 2022;**47**(7):582-595

[3] Deng J, Zhang T, Liu F, Han Q, Li Q, Guo X, et al. CRL4-DCAF8L2 E3 ligase promotes ubiquitination and degradation of BARD1. Biochemical and Biophysical Research Communications. 2022;**611**:107-113

[4] Russi M, Marson D, Fermeglia A, Aulic S, Fermeglia M, Laurini E, et al. The fellowship of the RING: BRCA1, its partner BARD1 and their liaison in DNA repair and cancer. Pharmacology & Therapeutics. 2022;**232**:108009

[5] Tarsounas M, Sung P. The antitumorigenic roles of BRCA1–BARD1 in DNA repair and replication. Nature Reviews Molecular Cell Biology. 2020;**21**(5):284-299

[6] Fox D et al. Crystal structure of the BARD1 ankyrin repeat domain and its functional consequences. The Journal of Biological Chemistry. 2008;**283**(30):21179-21186

[7] Yu X, Chini CCS, He M, Mer G, Chen J. The BRCT domain is a phosphoprotein binding domain. Science. 2003;**302**(5645):639-642

[8] Manke IA, Lowery DM, Nguyen A, Yaffe MB. BRCT repeats as phosphopeptide-binding modules involved in protein targeting. Science. 2003;**302**(5645):636-639

[9] Drost R, Bouwman P, Rottenberg S, Boon U, Schut E, Klarenbeek S, et al. BRCA1 RING function is essential for tumor suppression but dispensable for therapy resistance. Cancer Cell. 2011;**20**(6):797-809

[10] Shakya R, Reid LJ, Reczek CR, Cole F, Egli D, Lin C-S, et al. BRCA1 tumor suppression depends on BRCT phosphoprotein binding, but not its E3 ligase activity. Science. 2011;**334**(6055):525-528

[11] Fox D, Le Trong I, Rajagopal P, Brzovic PS, Stenkamp RE, Klevit RE. Crystal structure of the BARD1 ankyrin repeat domain and its functional consequences. Journal of Biological Chemistry. 2008;**283**(30):21179-21186

[12] Zhang YQ, Bianco A, Malkinson AM, Leoni VP, Frau G, De Rosa N, et al. BARD1: An independent predictor of survival in non-small cell lung cancer. International Journal of Cancer. 2012;**131**(1):83-94

[13] Ryser S, Dizin E, Jefford CE, Delaval B, Gagos S, Christodoulidou A, et al. Distinct roles of BARD1 isoforms in mitosis: Full-length BARD1 mediates Aurora B degradation, cancer-associated BARD1beta scaffolds Aurora B and BRCA2. Cancer Research. 2009;**69**(3):1125-1134

[14] Irminger-Finger I, Jefford CE. Is there more to BARD1 than BRCA1? Nature Reviews. Cancer. 2006;**6**(5):382-391

[15] Li L, Ryser S, Dizin E, Pils D, Krainer M, Jefford CE, et al. Oncogenic BARD1 isoforms expressed in gynecological cancers. Cancer Research. 2007;**67**(24):11876-11885

[16] Irminger-Finger I, Ratajska M, Pilyugin M. New concepts on BARD1: Regulator of BRCA pathways and beyond. The International Journal of Biochemistry & Cell Biology. 2016;**72**:1-17

[17] Cimmino F, Formicola D, Capasso M. Dualistic role of BARD1 in cancer. Genes. 2017;**8**(12):375

[18] Hawsawi YM, Al-Numair NS, Sobahy TM, Al-Ajmi AM, Al-Harbi RM, Baghdadi MA, et al. The role of BRCA1/2 in hereditary and familial breast and ovarian cancers. Molecular Genetics & Genomic Medicine. 2019;**7**(9):e879

[19] Alrefaei AF, Hawsawi YM, Almaleki D, Alafif T, Alzahrani FA, Bakhrebah MA. Genetic data sharing and artificial intelligence in the era of personalized medicine based on a cross-sectional analysis of the Saudi human genome program. Scientific Reports. 2022;**12**(1):1405

[20] Hawsawi YM, Shams A, Theyab A, Abdali WA, Hussien NA, Alatwi HE, et al. BARD1 mystery: Tumor suppressors are cancer susceptibility genes. BMC Cancer. 2022;**22**(1):599

[21] Jin Y, Xu XL, Yang MC, Wei F, Ayi TC, Bowcock AM, et al. Cell cycle-dependent colocalization of BARD1 and BRCA1 proteins in discrete nuclear domains. Proceedings of the National Academy of Sciences of the United States of America. 1997;**94**(22):12075-12080

[22] Scully R, Chen J, Ochs RL, Keegan K, Hoekstra M, Feunteun J, et al. Dynamic changes of BRCA1 subnuclear location and phosphorylation state are initiated by DNA damage. Cell. 1997;**90**(3):425-435

[23] Westermark UK, Reyngold M, Olshen AB, Baer R, Jasin M, Moynahan ME. BARD1 participates with BRCA1 in homology-directed repair of chromosome breaks. Molecular and Cellular Biology. 2003;**23**(21):7926-7936

[24] Li M, Yu X. Function of BRCA1 in the DNA damage response is mediated by ADP-ribosylation. Cancer Cell. 2013;**23**(5):693-704

[25] Billing D, Horiguchi M, Wu-Baer F, Taglialatela A, Leuzzi G, Nanez SA, et al. The BRCT domains of the BRCA1 and BARD1 tumor suppressors differentially regulate homology-directed repair and stalled fork protection. Molecular Cell. 2018;**72**(1):127-139

[26] Wu JY, Vlastos AT, Pelte MF, Caligo MA, Bianco A, Krause KH, et al. Aberrant expression of BARD1 in breast and ovarian cancers with poor prognosis. International Journal of Cancer. 2006;**118**(5):1215-1226

[27] Brzovic PS, Meza JE, King MC, Klevit RE. BRCA1 RING domain cancer-predisposing mutations. Structural consequences and effects on protein-protein interactions. The Journal of Biological Chemistry. 2001;**276**(44):41399-41406

[28] Thai TH, Du F, Tsan JT, Jin Y, Phung A, Spillman MA, et al. Mutations in the BRCA1-associated RING domain (BARD1) gene in primary breast, ovarian and uterine cancers. Human Molecular Genetics. 1998;**7**(2):195-202

[29] Ghimenti C, Sensi E, Presciuttini S, Brunetti IM, Conte P, Bevilacqua G, et al. Germline mutations of the BRCA1-associated ring domain (BARD1) gene in breast and breast/ovarian families negative for BRCA1 and BRCA2 alterations. Genes, Chromosomes & Cancer. 2002;**33**(3):235-242

[30] Ishitobi M, Miyoshi Y, Hasegawa S, Egawa C, Tamaki Y, Monden M, et al. Mutational analysis of BARD1 in familial

breast cancer patients in Japan. Cancer Letters. 2003;**200**(1):1-7

[31] Sedgwick SG, Smerdon SJ. The ankyrin repeat: A diversity of interactions on a common structural framework. Trends in Biochemical Sciences. 1999;**24**(8):311-316

[32] Kleiman FE, Manley JL. Functional interaction of BRCA1-associated BARD1 with polyadenylation factor CstF-50. Science. 1999;**285**(5433):1576-1579

[33] Kleiman FE, Manley JL. The BARD1-CstF-50 interaction links mRNA 3' end formation to DNA damage and tumor suppression. Cell. 2001;**104**(5):743-753

[34] Parvin JD. BRCA1 at a branch point. Proceedings of the National Academy of Sciences of the United States of America. 2001;**98**(11):5952-5954

[35] Fabbro M, Rodriguez JA, Baer R, Henderson BR. BARD1 induces BRCA1 intranuclear foci formation by increasing RING-dependent BRCA1 nuclear import and inhibiting BRCA1 nuclear export. The Journal of Biological Chemistry. 2002;**277**(24):21315-21324

[36] Irminger-Finger I, Leung WC, Li J, Dubois-Dauphin M, Harb J, Feki A, et al. Identification of BARD1 as mediator between proapoptotic stress and p53-dependent apoptosis. Molecular Cell. 2001;**8**(6):1255-1266

[37] Dechend R, Hirano F, Lehmann K, Heissmeyer V, Ansieau S, Wulczyn FG, et al. The Bcl-3 oncoprotein acts as a bridging factor between NF-kappaB/Rel and nuclear co-regulators. Oncogene. 1999;**18**(22):3316-3323

[38] Irminger-Finger I, Soriano JV, Vaudan G, Montesano R, Sappino AP. In vitro repression of Brca1-associated RING domain gene, Bard1, induces phenotypic changes in mammary epithelial cells. The Journal of Cell Biology. 1998;**143**(5):1329-1339

[39] McCarthy EE, Celebi JT, Baer R, Ludwig T. Loss of Bard1, the heterodimeric partner of the Brca1 tumor suppressor, results in early embryonic lethality and chromosomal instability. Molecular and Cellular Biology. 2003;**23**(14):5056-5063

[40] Dizin E, Irminger-Finger I. Negative feedback loop of BRCA1–BARD1 ubiquitin ligase on estrogen receptor alpha stability and activity antagonized by cancer-associated isoform of BARD1. The International Journal of Biochemistry & Cell Biology. 2010;**42**(5):693-700

[41] Śniadecki M, Brzeziński M, Darecka K, Klasa-Mazurkiewicz D, Poniewierza P, Krzeszowiec M, et al. Bard1 and breast cancer: The possibility of creating screening tests and new preventive and therapeutic pathways for predisposed women. Genes. 2020;**11**(11):1251

[42] Norquist BM, Harrell MI, Brady MF, Walsh T, Lee MK, Gulsuner S, et al. Inherited mutations in women with ovarian carcinoma. JAMA Oncology. 2016;**2**(4):482-490

[43] Couch FJ, Shimelis H, Hu C, Hart SN, Polley EC, Na J, et al. Associations between cancer predisposition testing panel genes and breast cancer. JAMA Oncology. 2017;**3**(9):1190-1196

[44] Sporn JC, Hothorn T, Jung B. BARD1 expression predicts outcome in colon cancer. Clinical Cancer Research. 2011;**17**(16):5451-5462

[45] Ozden O, Bishehsari F, Bauer J, Park SH, Jana A, Baik SH, et al. Expression of an oncogenic BARD1

splice variant impairs homologous recombination and predicts response to PARP-1 inhibitor therapy in colon cancer. Scientific Reports. 2016;**6**:26273

[46] Lepore I, Dell'Aversana C, Pilyugin M, Conte M, Nebbioso A, De Bellis F, et al. HDAC inhibitors repress BARD1 isoform expression in acute myeloid leukemia cells via activation of miR-19a and/or b. PLoS One. 2013;**8**(12):e83018

[47] Creekmore AL, Ziegler YS, Bonéy JL, Nardulli AM. Estrogen receptor α regulates expression of the breast cancer 1 associated ring domain 1 (BARD1) gene through intronic DNA sequence. Molecular and Cellular Endocrinology. 2007;**267**(1-2):106-115

[48] Hu WL, Jin L, Xu A, Wang YF, Thorne RF, Zhang XD, et al. GUARDIN is a p53-responsive long non-coding RNA that is essential for genomic stability. Nature Cell Biology. 2018;**20**(4):492-502

[49] Xu Y, Wang Y, Luo J, Zhao W, Zhou X. Deep learning of the splicing (epi) genetic code reveals a novel candidate mechanism linking histone modifications to ESC fate decision. Nucleic Acids Research. 2017;**45**(21):12100-12112

[50] Watters AK, Seltzer ES, MacKenzie D, Young M, Muratori J, Hussein R, et al. The effects of genetic and epigenetic alterations of BARD1 on the development of non-breast and non-gynecological cancers. Genes. 2020;**11**(7):829

[51] Huber-Keener KJ. Cancer genetics and breast cancer. Clinical Obstetrics & Gynaecology. 2022;**82**:3-11

[52] Alzahrani FA, Ahmed F, Sharma M, Rehan M, Mahfuz M, Baeshen MN, et al. Investigating the pathogenic SNPs in BLM helicase and their biological consequences by computational approach. Scientific Reports. 2020;**10**(1):12377

[53] Alzahrani FA, Hawsawi YM, Altayeb HN, Alsiwiehri NO, Alzahrani OR, Alatwi HE, et al. In silico modeling of the interaction between TEX19 and LIRE1, and analysis of TEX19 gene missense SNPs. Molecular Genetics & Genomic Medicine. 2021;**2021**:e1707

[54] Barnawi I, Hawsawi Y, Dash P, Oyouni AAA, Mustafa SK, Hussien NA, et al. Nitric oxide synthase potentiates the resistance of cancer cell lines to anticancer chemotherapeutics. Anti-Cancer Agents in Medicinal Chemistry. 2022;**22**(7):1397-1406(10)

[55] Kotb A, El Fakih R, Hanbali A, Hawsawi Y, Alfraih F, Hashmi S, et al. Philadelphia-like acute lymphoblastic leukemia: Diagnostic dilemma and management perspectives. Experimental Hematology. 2018;**67**:1-9

[56] Hawsawi YM, Zailaie SA, Oyouni AAA, Alzahrani OR, Alamer OM, Aljohani SAS. Prostate cancer and therapeutic challenges. Journal of Biological Research (Thessaloniki). 2020;**27**(1):20

[57] Yamamoto H, Hirasawa A. Homologous recombination deficiencies and hereditary tumors. International Journal of Molecular Sciences. 2022;**23**(1):348

[58] Semlali A, Almutairi M, Rouabhia M, Reddy Parine N, Al Amri A. Novel sequence variants in the TLR6 gene associated with advanced breast cancer risk in the Saudi Arabian population. PLoS One. 2018;**13**(11):2033

[59] Alanazi IO, Shaik JP, Parine NR, Azzam NA, Alharbi O, Hawsawi YM, et al. Association of HER1 and HER2 Gene Variants in the Predisposition of

Colorectal Cancer. Journal of Oncology. 2021;**2021**:6180337

[60] Thirumal Kumar D, Kumar SU, Jain N, Sowmya B, Balsekar K, Siva R, et al. Computational structural assessment of BReast CAncer type 1 susceptibility protein (BRCA1) and BRCA1-Associated Ring Domain protein 1 (BARD1) mutations on the protein-protein interface. Advances in Protein Chemistry and Structural Biology. 2022;**130**:375-397

[61] Peto J, Collins N, Barfoot R, Seal S, Warren W, Rahman N, et al. Prevalence of BRCA1 and BRCA2 gene mutations in patients with early-onset breast cancer. Journal of the National Cancer Institute. 1999;**91**(11):943-949

[62] Shiovitz S, Korde LA. Genetics of breast cancer: A topic in evolution. Annals of Oncology. 2015;**26**(7):1291-1299

[63] Michailidou K, Lindström S, Dennis J, Beesley J, Hui S, Kar S, et al. Association analysis identifies 65 new breast cancer risk loci. Nature. 2017;**551**(7678):92-94

[64] Li W, Gu X, Liu C, Shi Y, Wang P, Zhang N, et al. A synergetic effect of BARD1 mutations on tumorigenesis. Nature Communications. 2021;**12**(1):1-13

[65] Thai TH, Du F, Tsan JT, Jin Y, Phung A, Spillman MA, et al. Mutations in the BRCAI-associated RING d(BARD1) gene in primary breast, ovarian and uterine cancers. Human Molecular Genetics. 1998;**7**(2):195-202

[66] Huo X, Hu Z, Zhai X, Wang Y, Wang S, Wang X, et al. Common non-synonymous polymorphisms in the BRCA1 Associated RING Domain (BARD1) gene are associated with breast cancer susceptibility: A case-control analysis. Breast Cancer Research and Treatment. 2007;**102**(3):329-337

[67] Suszynska M, Kluzniak W, WokolorczykD,JakubowskaA,HuzarskiT, Gronwald J, et al. Bard1 is a low/moderate breast cancer risk gene: Evidence based on an association study of the central European p. q564x recurrent mutation. Cancer. 2019;**11**(6):740

[68] Shimelis H, LaDuca H, Hu C, Hart SN, Na J, Thomas A, et al. Triple-negative breast cancer risk genes identified by multigene hereditary cancer panel testing. Journal of the National Cancer Institute. 2018;**110**(8):855-862

[69] Wu J, Aini A, Ma B. Mutations in exon region of BRCA1-related RING domain 1 gene and risk of breast cancer. Molecular Genetics & Genomic Medicine. 2022;**2022**:e1847

[70] Suszynska M, Kozlowski P. Summary of bard1 mutations and precise estimation of breast and ovarian cancer risks associated with the mutations. Genes. 2020;**11**(7):798

[71] Stewart MD, Zelin E, Dhall A, Walsh T, Upadhyay E, Corn JE, et al. BARD1 is necessary for ubiquitylation of nucleosomal histone H2A and for transcriptional regulation of estrogen metabolism genes. Proceedings of the National Academy of Sciences of the United States of America. 2018;**115**(6):1316-1321

[72] Adamovich AI, Banerjee T, Wingo M, Duncan K, Ning J, Martins Rodrigues F, et al. Functional analysis of BARD1 missense variants in homology-directed repair and damage sensitivity. PLoS Genetics. 2019;**15**(3):e1008049

[73] Zheng Y, Li B, Pan D, Cao J, Zhang J, Wang X, et al. Functional consequences of a rare missense BARD1 c. 403G> A germline mutation identified in a triple-negative breast cancer patient. Breast Cancer Research. 2021;**23**(1):1-7

[74] Bosse KR, Diskin SJ, Cole KA, Wood AC, Schnepp RW, Norris G, et al. Common variation at BARD1 results in the expression of an oncogenic isoform that influences neuroblastoma susceptibility and oncogenicity. Cancer Research. 2012;**72**(8):2068-2078

[75] Karppinen SM, Heikkinen K, Rapakko K, Winqvist R. Mutation screening of the BARD1 gene: Evidence for involvement of the Cys557Ser allele in hereditary susceptibility to breast cancer. Journal of Medical Genetics. 2004;**41**(9):e114

[76] Fu W, Zhu J, Xiong S-W, Jia W, Zhao Z, Zhu S-B, et al. BARD1 gene polymorphisms confer nephroblastoma susceptibility. eBioMedicine. 2017;**16**:101-105

[77] Shi J, Yu Y, Jin Y, Lu J, Zhang J, Wang H, et al. Functional polymorphisms in BARD1 association with neuroblastoma in a regional Han Chinese population. Journal of Cancer. 2019;**10**(10):2153

[78] Feki A, Jefford CE, Berardi P, Wu JY, Cartier L, Krause KH, et al. BARD1 induces apoptosis by catalysing phosphorylation of p53 by DNA-damage response kinase. Oncogene. 2005;**24**(23):3726-3736

[79] Walsh T, Casadei S, Lee MK, Pennil CC, Nord AS, Thornton AM, et al. Mutations in 12 genes for inherited ovarian, fallopian tube, and peritoneal carcinoma identified by massively parallel sequencing. Proceedings of the National Academy of Sciences of the United States of America. 2011;**108**(44):18032-18037

[80] Ratajska M, Antoszewska E, Piskorz A, Brozek I, Borg A, Kusmierek H, et al. Cancer predisposing BARD1 mutations in breast-ovarian cancer families. Breast Cancer Research and Treatment. 2012;**131**(1):89-97

[81] Pennington KP, Walsh T, Harrell MI, Lee MK, Pennil CC, Rendi MH, et al. Germline and somatic mutations in homologous recombination genes predict platinum response and survival in ovarian, fallopian tube, and peritoneal carcinomas. Clinical Cancer Research. 2014;**20**(3):764-775

[82] Stacey SN, Sulem P, Johannsson OT, Helgason A, Gudmundsson J, Kostic JP, et al. The BARD1 Cys557Ser variant and breast cancer risk in Iceland. PLoS Medicine. 2006;**3**(7):e217

[83] Gonzalez-Hormazabal P, Reyes JM, Blanco R, Bravo T, Carrera I, Peralta O, et al. The BARD1 Cys557Ser variant and risk of familial breast cancer in a South-American population. Molecular Biology Reports. 2012;**39**(8):8091-8098

[84] Johnatty SE, Beesley J, Chen X, Hopper JL, Southey MC, Giles GG, et al. The BARD1 Cys557Ser polymorphism and breast cancer risk: An Australian case–control and family analysis. Breast Cancer Research and Treatment. 2009;**115**(1):145-150

[85] Vahteristo P, Syrjäkoski K, Heikkinen T, Eerola H, Aittomäki K, von Smitten K, et al. BARD1 variants Cys557Ser and Val507Met in breast cancer predisposition. European Journal of Human Genetics. 2006;**14**(2):167-172

[86] Jakubowska A, Cybulski C, Szymańska A, Huzarski T, Byrski T, Gronwald J, et al. BARD1 and breast cancer in Poland. Breast Cancer Research and Treatment. 2008;**107**(1):119-122

[87] Gorringe KL, Choong DY, Visvader JE, Lindeman GJ, Campbell IG. BARD1 variants are not associated with breast cancer risk in Australian familial

breast cancer. Breast Cancer Research and Treatment. 2008;**111**(3):505-509

[88] Spurdle AB, Marquart L, McGuffog L, Healey S, Sinilnikova O, Wan F, et al. Common genetic variation at BARD1 is not associated with breast cancer risk in BRCA1 or BRCA2 mutation carriers. Cancer Epidemiology and Prevention Biomarkers. 2011;**20**(5):1032-1038

[89] Zhu Y, Liu Y, Zhang C, Chu J, Wu Y, Li Y, et al. Tamoxifen-resistant breast cancer cells are resistant to DNA-damaging chemotherapy because of upregulated BARD1 and BRCA1. Nature Communications. 2018;**9**(1):1595

[90] Maximov PY, Abderrahman B, Hawsawi YM, Chen Y, Foulds CE, Jain A, et al. The structure-function relationship of angular estrogens and estrogen receptor alpha to initiate estrogen-induced apoptosis in breast cancer cells. Molecular Pharmacology. 2020;**98**(1):24-37

[91] Jordan VC, Fan P, Abderrahman B, Maximov PY, Hawsawi YM, Bhattacharya P, et al. Sex steroid induced apoptosis as a rational strategy to treat anti-hormone resistant breast and prostate cancer. Discovery Medicine. 2016;**21**(117):411-427

[92] Hawsawi Y, El-Gendy R, Twelves C, Speirs V, Beattie J. Insulin-like growth factor – oestradiol crosstalk and mammary gland tumourigenesis. Biochimica et Biophysica Acta. 2013;**1836**(2):345-353

[93] Watanabe Y, Maeda I, Oikawa R, Wu W, Tsuchiya K, Miyoshi Y, et al. Aberrant DNA methylation status of DNA repair genes in breast cancer treated with neoadjuvant chemotherapy. Genes to Cells. 2013;**18**(12):1120-1130

[94] Gonzalez-Rivera M, Lobo M, Lopez-Tarruella S, Jerez Y, Del Monte-Millan M, Massarrah T, et al. Frequency of germline DNA genetic findings in an unselected prospective cohort of triple-negative breast cancer patients participating in a platinum-based neoadjuvant chemotherapy trial. Breast Cancer Research and Treatment. 2016;**156**(3):507-515

[95] Post AEM, Bussink J, Sweep F, Span PN. Changes in DNA damage repair gene expression and cell cycle gene expression do not explain radioresistance in tamoxifen-resistant breast cancer. Oncology Research. 2020;**28**(1):33-40

[96] Hawsawi Y, Humphries MP, Wright A, Berwick A, Shires M, Al-Kharobi H, et al. Deregulation of IGF-binding proteins -2 and -5 contributes to the development of endocrine resistant breast cancer in vitro. Oncotarget. 2016;**7**(22):32129-32143

[97] Ledermann J, Harter P, Gourley C, Friedlander M, Vergote I, Rustin G, et al. Olaparib maintenance therapy in patients with platinum-sensitive relapsed serous ovarian cancer: A preplanned retrospective analysis of outcomes by BRCA status in a randomised phase 2 trial. The Lancet Oncology. 2014;**15**(8):852-861

Section 4

BRCA-Associated Cancers

Chapter 5

BRCA Gene Mutations and Prostate Cancer

Gvantsa Kharaishvili, Mariam Kacheishvili and Giorgi Akhvlediani

Abstract

Prostate cancer remains the second most common cancer in men, with diverse courses from indolent cases to aggressive diseases. Among the key factors implicated in its pathogenesis are genomic alterations such as the TMPRSS2-ERG and related fusion oncogenes, loss of tumor suppressor PTEN, p53 or NKX3.1, inflammation, enhanced DNA damage, and chromosomal instability. Men with prostate cancer who carry BRCA1/2 mutations are at more risk of worse disease and poor prognosis. Cancer cells with mutant BRCA1 or BRCA2 repair genes with defects in homologous recombination are vulnerable to PARP inhibitors that target the genetic phenomenon known as synthetic lethality to exploit faulty DNA repair mechanisms. With relevance to prostate cancer, other features of cancer cells may also sensitize to PARP inhibitors, including aberrant transcription due to the androgen-driven fusion oncogene TMPRSS2-ERG or PTEN loss. Several models of synthetic lethality and potential biomarkers suggested up to date are also discussed. The chapter also highlights the importance of genetic screening of men with BRCA and shows diagnostic utility of plasma-derived circulating tumor DNA.

Keywords: prostate cancer, metastatic disease, BRCA1, BRCA2, PARPi, biomarkers

1. Introduction

Prostate cancer is one of the most common malignancies in men and a significant cause of cancer-related deaths [1]. Its incidence varies between less to highly developed countries with highlights of the implication of diagnostic practices, mainly PSA screening and lifestyle and environmental risk factors [2]. A family history of the disease is also a well-stated risk factor for prostate cancer. The risk for first-degree relatives of men with prostate cancer is about twice that for men in the general population [3]. Like all cancers, prostate cancer is a genetic disease driven by the activation of oncogenes as well as the depression of tumor suppressors [2]. The cross talk between multiple genes and environmental factors results in complex molecular pathogenesis in the development of prostate cancer (PCa), and these genetic and epigenetic changes can develop at various stages. Prostate cancer has multiple genetic alterations, including somatic copy number or chromosomal number changes, point mutations, and various structural modifications [4]. Somatic copy number alterations may be found in around 90% of PCa cases. Primary PCa often shows deletions on different chromosome numbers such as 6q, 8p, 10q, and 13q. In metastatic castration-resistant prostate cancer (mCRPC), the augmentation of chromosomes x, 7, 8q, and 9q has been identified [5]. Genes related to prostate cancer development and their chromosomal localization are summarized in a review by Kral and colleagues [6]. Hereditary prostate cancer (HPCa) has the highest heritability of any cancer in men. The proportion of PCa attributable to hereditary factors has been estimated at 5–15%. To date, the genes more consistently associated with HPCa susceptibility include mismatch repair (MMR) genes (MLH1, MSH2, MSH6, and PMS2) and homologous recombination genes (e.g., BRCA1 and BRCA2, ATM, PALB2, or CHEK2). Additional genes should be integrated into specific research, including HOXB13, BRP1, and NSB1 [7–9]. BRCA1 and BRCA2, together with PALB2 or BARD1, are critical mediators of the HRR process, and their loss results in functional impairment of the HRR pathway [10].

2. Current challenges in prostate cancer research and treatment

Significant advances have been made in understanding prostate cancer's molecular makeup, diagnosis, and treatment, e.g., approval of novel drugs that improve survival in men with advanced prostate cancer. Nonetheless, several areas of unmet need remain, for example, adjuvant therapies to increase cure rates in higher-risk locally advanced diseases or treatment of metastatic cancer [3]. Novel therapeutic strategies tailored to biologically defined prostate cancer subsets are being developed thanks to clinical trial benefits, new drugs, the use of NGS, advanced functional imaging, and the better use of existing therapies in early-stage disease [3]. PCa initiation and progression are driven by androgen receptor (AR) signaling. PCa is uniquely dependent on androgens for growth and progression, and androgen deprivation therapy (ADT) is an effective treatment for patients with advanced disease. However, when a castration-resistant state develops, the patient has more chance of dying of PCa than other causes. Alterations in AR signaling in metastatic castration-resistant PCa (mCRPC) include persistent AR activation, which leads to AR amplification, AR splice variants, and intratumoral androgen biosynthesis. Enzalutamide, an AR antagonist, blocks AR translocation function, and Abiraterone inhibits androgen biosynthesis [7]. Recently, mCRPC patients with germline defects in DNA damage repair showed a decreased response to AR-targeted therapy. At the same time, other authors reported an improved response to second-generation ADT with the administration of drugs, including Abiraterone or Enzalutamide, in men with BRCA or ATM mutations [7].

3. BRCA1 and BRCA2 importance in prostate cancer

BRCA1 and BRCA2 genes are inherited in an autosomal dominant manner. Men and women have an equal chance of inheriting either of these genes and passing them to their descendants. There are numerous studies investigating the cancer risks and outcomes of female carriers, while studies of the cancer characteristics in male carriers are still lacking [11]. Men with germline BRCA1 and BRCA2 mutations are less investigated than female peers [11]. The risk of breast cancer in BRCA1 carrier men at age 70 is 1.2%, while for BRCA2 carriers is 6.8%. Besides breast cancer, male germline mutation carriers also have an increased lifetime risk for prostate cancer with a cumulative lifetime risk of 29% (95% CI = 17–45%) for BRCA1-mutation carriers and 60% (95% CI = 43–78%) for BRCA2-mutation carriers compared with a lifetime risk of 16% of the general population [12, 13]. Familial aggregation of mutations is also well documented in Laitinen et al. [14]. Men with a family history of prostate cancer in first-degree relatives bear an increased risk of the disease, as shown in a long-term follow-up study among Nordic twins [15]. The Prostate Cancer database Sweden (PCBaSE) study also confirmed a 14.9% risk of developing prostate cancer in men of age 65, compared with 4.8% for men who did not have a brother with prostate cancer. At age 75, the risk of developing prostate cancer was 30.3% for patients having a brother with the disease vs. 12.9% for patients without a brother with PCa [16].

The clinical impact of the role of DNA damage repair genes is still evolving in PCa, although it likely mirrors the path of hereditary breast and ovarian cancer [8]. Transformations in BRCA1 and BRCA2 have recognized the factor for the progression of poor-risk PCa. Besides BRCA1 and BRCA2, cancer cells with mutant BRCA1 or BRCA2 repair genes with defects in homologous recombination are vulnerable to poly (ADP-ribose) polymerase (PARP) inhibitors that target the genetic phenomenon known as synthetic lethality to exploit faulty DNA repair mechanisms.

The notion of synthetic lethality stems from genetic studies on the fruit fly Drosophila Melanogaster [17]. It describes the example of the co-occurrence of different gene mutations resulting in cell death where an individual, single genetic event is still compatible with life [18]. Unlike conventional targeted drugs, synthetic lethal therapy promotes indirect mutation targeting by identifying an alternative synthetic lethal target that may include oncogenes, tumor suppressors, DNA repair machinery, cancer metabolism agents, etc. [19]. Synthetic lethal relationships can potentially broaden the strategies of novel anticancer treatments. Identification and validation of potential synthetic lethal partner genes represent the challenge of current research. Clinical studies on breast cancer BRCA carriers described the auspicious synthetic lethal effect of BRCA/PARP [20]. Later, several mechanisms of resistance to PARP inhibitors were suggested. These are secondary mutations of BRCA1 and BRCA2, as well as upregulation of the gene encoding P-glycoprotein pump or loss of TP53BP1 protein [20].

4. Prognostic role of BRCA mutations in prostate cancer

The largest comprehensive study of clinicopathologic, therapeutic, and survival data of 2181 prostate cancer patients was processed to evaluate the evidence for the independent prognostic value of BRCA1/2 mutation status on PCa cause-specific survival (CSS). Patients cohorts included in study were from United Kingdom Genetic Prostate Cancer study (UKGPCS) and Epidemiological Study of BRCA1/2 Mutation Carriers (EMBRACE). The Study showed that node involvement and distant metastasis are more common in patients with PCa who have BRCA1/2 mutations and those carriers with local disease develop metastasis earlier [21]. Further, poor outcome was mostly dependent on BRCA2, whereas the contribution of BRCA1 mutations remained unclear [21]. Taken together, BRCA1/2 mutations are associated with a more aggressive disease/lethal prostate cancer and the proportion of germline mutations in localized disease is 4.6% while 11.8–16.2% is observed in metastatic cases [22]. Presence of such a mutations, however, also identifies individuals who could benefit from PARP inhibitors [23]. Moreover, presence of BRCA mutations can predict response to drugs based on platinum salts [24]. Other HRR mutations are also frequent, but their prognostic/predictive importance for prostate cancer patients remains elusive. Moreover, a proportion of these mutations are associated with inherited germline defects and are relevant to the patients' risk of second malignancies and their relatives' risk of cancer [10].

5. Importance of genetic screening of men with BRCA

The character of available information on BRCA1/2-related cancers is directed mainly at women, reflecting a gendered approach that may lead men to underestimate their risk of carrying BRCA mutations [25]. The determinants of men's motivations to engage in genetic screening for BRCA1 and BRCA2 were explored in a very recent study by Annoni and Longhini [26] through the lens of the Health Action Process Approach. One-hundred and twenty-five men with a mean age of 58.53 ± 10.37 participated in an online survey. The intention to undergo genetic screening for BRCA1/2 mutations in men was significantly and positively associated with self-efficacy and risk perception. Moreover, having offspring positively affected intention as well. Petrylak et al. [27] highlighted the importance of genomic screening as part of a comprehensive assessment of prostate cancer prognosis and treatment options and suggested plasma as the best material to select patients with mCRPC for treatment with a PARP inhibitor [27]. The authors noted that the analysis of plasma and archival biopsy samples obtained before the patient started Rucaparib treatment detected the same alterations. However, BRCA2 homozygous loss (whole gene, 26 of 26 exons) and several other alterations were also detected, but in plasma only. Authors hypothesize that the response of the patient's tumor to Rucaparib was likely driven by DNA damage repair deficiency caused by homozygous loss of all BRCA2 exons [27]. A similar approach was suggested by Chi and colleagues [28], when evaluating the utility of plasma-derived circulating tumor DNA (ctDNA) in identifying BRCA1, BRCA2, and ATM alterations in patients with mCRPC from the phase III PROfound study. They showed that 81% of ctDNA samples yielded an NGS result. BRCA and ATM status in tissue compared with ctDNA showed 81% positive percentage agreement and 92% negative percentage agreement when tissue was a reference. The concordance was high for nonsense (93%), splice (87%), and frameshift (86%) mutations but lower for large rearrangements (63%) and homozygous deletions (27%) [28].

6. Therapeutic targeting of men with BRCA1 and BRCA2 mutations

The mutation status of genes involved in PCa may impact therapeutic strategies. PARP inhibitors such as Olaparib, Rucaparib, Niraparib, and Telazoparib, effectively kill tumors defective in the BRCA1 or BRCA2 genes through the concept of synthetic lethality, causing selective tumor cell cytotoxicity in cell lines [29]. According to one suggested model, PARP inhibitors cause an increase in DNA single-strand breaks (SSBs), which, during replication, are converted to irreparable toxic DNA double-strand breaks (DSBs) in BRCA1/2 defective cells. Alternative models suggested by Helleday [29] are not mutually exclusive. One of the models proposes that PARP inhibition causes PARP-1 to be trapped onto DNA repair intermediates during base excision repair. This may, in turn, obstruct replication forks, which require BRCA-dependent homologous recombination to be resolved [29]. According to another model, PARP is directly involved in catalyzing replication repair in a distinct pathway from homologous recombination. Targeting DNA repair defects by PARP1 inhibitors requires suitable predictive biomarkers. The third phase of the clinical trial was conducted on two groups of men having alterations in genes involved in homologous recombination repair with progressing metastatic castration-resistant prostate cancer while receiving Enzalutamide or Abiraterone: Cohort A with at least one alteration in BRCA1, BRCA2, or ATM, and cohort B with alterations in any of 12 other prespecified genes. Olaparib was associated with more prolonged progression-free survival and better response measures and patient-reported endpoints than either enzalutamide or Abiraterone [30]. Kurfurstova et al. [31] performed an immunohistochemical analysis of multiple markers of DNA damage signaling, oxidative stress, DNA repair, and cell cycle control pathways in human prostate benign hyperplasia, intraepithelial neoplasia, and PCa and observed that the DNA damage checkpoint barrier (γH2AX, pATM, p53) mechanism was activated during PCa tumorigenesis. The authors observed that oxidative stress (8-Oxoguanine lesions) and NQO1 increased during disease progression.

Interestingly, TMPRSS2-ERG rearrangement and PTEN loss are events sensitizing to PARPi, frequently occurring along with heterogeneous loss of DNA repair factors 53BP1, JMJD1C, and Rev7. Their defects may cause resistance to PARPi [31]. Oplustilova et al. [32] evaluate several other biomarkers, such as spontaneous PARsylation and Rad51 foci formation, as surrogate markers for PARP activity and HR, respectively, supporting their candidacy for biomarkers of PARP-1i responses [32]. Altmeyer [33], in its comment on the research article by Oplustilova ct al. [32], mentions that the use of single biomarkers could indeed be misleading and that a combination of markers to assess which cancer cells are likely "addicted to PAR" might be more reliable [33].

7. Concluding remarks and perspectives

BRCA1 and BRCA2 tumor suppressors gained higher clinical significance with regard to metastatic and lethal prostate cancer. BRCA2 was demonstrated as a strong predictor of response to PARP inhibitors. Molecular characterization of mCRPC patients should be integrated into routine clinical testing to select potential responders to treatment. This chapter contributes to the role of BRCA1 and BRCA2 gene alterations in prostate cancer. A more detailed understanding of the complex DNA damage repair network in prostate cancer with an unstable genome will give deeper insights into the diverse functions of PARPs and potential contributors of synthetic lethality.

Author details

Gvantsa Kharaishvili[1,2,3*], Mariam Kacheishvili[3] and Giorgi Akhvlediani[4,5]

1 Faculty of Medicine and Dentistry, Department of Clinical and Molecular Pathology, Palacky University, Czech Republic

2 Faculty Hospital in Olomouc, Olomouc, Czech Republic

3 David Tvildiani Medical University, Tbilisi, Georgia

4 Georgian-American University, Tbilisi, Georgia

5 American Hospital in Tbilisi, Tbilisi, Georgia

*Address all correspondence to: gvantsa.kharaishvili@upol.cz

References

[1] Available from: https://www.wcrf.org/cancer-trends/prostate-cancer-statistics

[2] WHO. WHO Classification of Tumours of the Urinary System and Male Genital Organs. Lyon, France: International Agency for Research on Cancer; 2016

[3] Attard G, Parker C, Eeles RA, et al. Prostate cancer. Lancet. 2016;**387**(10013):70-82. DOI: 10.1016/S0140-6736(14)61947-4

[4] Schoenborn JR, Nelson P, Fang M. Genomic profiling defines subtypes of prostate cancer with the potential for therapeutic stratification. Clinical Cancer Research. 2013;**19**(15):4058-4066. DOI: 10.1158/1078-0432.CCR-12-3606

[5] Junejo NN, AlKhateeb SS. BRCA2 gene mutation and prostate cancer risk. Comprehensive review and update. Saudi Medical Journal. 2020;**41**(1):9-17. DOI: 10.15537/smj.2020.1.24759

[6] Kral M, Rosinska V, Student V, Grepl M, Hrabec M, Bouchal J. Genetic determinants of prostate cancer: A review. Biomedical Papers of the Medical Faculty of the University Palacky, Olomouc, Czech Republic. 2011;**155**(1):3-9. DOI: 10.5507/bp.155.2011.001

[7] Vietri MT, D'Elia G, Caliendo G, Resse M, Casamassimi A, Passariello L, et al. Hereditary prostate cancer: Genes related, target therapy and prevention. International Journal of Molecular Sciences. 2021;**22**:3753. DOI: 10.3390/ijms22073753

[8] Das S, Salami SS, Spratt DE, Kaffenberger SD, Jacobs MF, Morgan TM. Bringing prostate cancer germline genetics into clinical practice. The Journal of Urology. 2019;**202**(2):223-230. DOI: 10.1097/JU.0000000000000137

[9] Pritchard CC, Offit K, Nelson PS. DNA-repair gene mutations in metastatic prostate cancer. The New England Journal of Medicine. 2016;**375**(18):1804-1805. DOI: 10.1056/NEJMc1611137

[10] Cresta Morgado P, Mateo J. Clinical implications of homologous recombination repair mutations in prostate cancer. The Prostate. 2022;**82**:S45-S59. DOI: 10.1002/pros.24352

[11] Reichl F, Muhr D, Rebhan K, et al. Cancer spectrum, family history of cancer and overall survival in men with germline BRCA1 or BRCA2 mutations. Journal of Persian Medicine. 2021;**11**(9):917

[12] Mahon SM. Cancer risks for men with BRCA1/2 mutations. Oncology Nursing Forum. 2014;**41**(1):99-101. DOI: 10.1188/14.ONF.99-101

[13] Moran A, O'Hara C, Khan S, et al. Risk of cancer other than breast or ovarian in individuals with BRCA1 and BRCA2 mutations. Familial Cancer. 2012;**11**(2):235-242. DOI: 10.1007/s10689-011-9506-2

[14] Laitinen VH, Akinrinade O, Rantapero T, Tammela TL, Wahlfors T, Schleutker J. Germline copy number variation analysis in Finnish families with hereditary prostate cancer. The Prostate. 2016;**76**(3):316-324. DOI: 10.1002/pros.23123

[15] Mucci LA, Hjelmborg JB, Harris JR, Czene K, Havelick DJ, Scheike T, et al. Familial risk and heritability of cancer among twins in Nordic countries. JAMA. 2016;**315**(8):822

[16] Bratt O, Drevin L, Akre O, Garmo H, Stattin P. Family history and probability of prostate cancer, differentiated by risk category: A nationwide population-based study. Journal of the National Cancer Institute. 2016;**108**(10):djw110

[17] Lucchesi JC. Synthetic lethality and semi-lethality among functionally related mutants of *Drosophila melanogaster*. Genetics. 1968;**59**(1):37-44. DOI: 10.1093/genetics/59.1.37

[18] Iglehart JD, Silver DP. Synthetic lethality—A new direction in cancer-drug development. The New England Journal of Medicine. 2009;**361**(2):189-191

[19] O'Neil NJ, Bailey ML, Hieter P. Synthetic lethality and cancer. Nature Reviews. Genetics. 2017;**18**(10):613-623

[20] Bouchalova K, Hajduch M. Prediktivní a Prognostická Onkologie. Univerzita Palackho v Olomouci. 2016.

[21] Castro E, Goh C, Olmos D, Saunders E, Leongamornlert D, Tymrakiewicz M, et al. Germline BRCA mutations are associated with higher risk of nodal involvement, distant metastasis, and poor survival outcomes in prostate cancer. Journal of Clinical Oncology. 2013;**31**(14):1748-1757. DOI: 10.1200/JCO.2012.43

[22] McNevin CS, Cadoo K, Baird AM, Murchan P, Sheils O, McDermott R, et al. Pathogenic BRCA variants as biomarkers for risk in prostate cancer. Cancers (Basel). 2021;**13**(22):5697. DOI: 10.3390/cancers13225697

[23] Mateo J, Carreira S, Sandhu S, Miranda S, Mossop H, Perez-Lopez R, et al. DNA-repair defects and olaparib in metastatic prostate cancer. The New England Journal of Medicine. 2015;**373**(18):1697-1708. DOI: 10.1056/NEJMoa1506859

[24] Pomerantz MM, Spisák S, Jia L, Cronin AM, Csabai I, Ledet E, et al. The association between germline BRCA2 variants and sensitivity to platinum-based chemotherapy among men with metastatic prostate cancer. Cancer. 2017;**123**(18):3532-3539. DOI: 10.1002/cncr.30808

[25] Thomas E. Original research: Men's awareness and knowledge of male breast cancer. The American Journal of Nursing. 2010;**110**(10):32-42. DOI: 10.1097/01.NAJ.0000389672.93605.2f

[26] Annoni AM, Longhini C. Investigating men's motivations to engage in genetic screening for BRCA1 and BRCA2 mutations. PLoS One. 2022;**17**(3):e0265387. DOI: 10.1371/journal.pone.0265387

[27] Petrylak DP, Watkins SP, Loehr A. What plasma can tell us when tissue cannot: A case report of genomic testing in mCRPC and clinical response to treatment with the PARP inhibitor rucaparib. Frontier in Oncologia. 2022;**12**:951348

[28] Chi KN, Barnicle A, Sibilla C, et al. Detection of BRCA1, BRCA2, and ATM alterations in matched tumor tissue and circulating tumor DNA in patients with prostate cancer screened in PROfound. Clinical Cancer Research. 2022;**2022**:OF1-OF11. DOI: 10.1158/1078-0432.CCR-22-0931

[29] Helleday T. The underlying mechanism for the PARP and BRCA synthetic lethality: Clearing up the misunderstandings. Molecular Oncology. 2011;5(4):387-393

[30] de Bono J, Mateo J, Fizazi K, Saad F, Shore N, Sandhu S, et al. Olaparib for metastatic castration-resistant prostate cancer. The New England Journal of Medicine. 2020;**382**(22):2091-2102

[31] Kurfurstova D, Bartkova J, Vrtel R, Mickova A, Burdova A, Majera D, et al. DNA damage signalling barrier, oxidative stress and treatment-relevant DNA repair factor alterations during progression of human prostate cancer. Molecular Oncology. 2016;**10**(6):879-894. DOI: 10.1016/j.molonc.2016.02.005

[32] Oplustilova L, Wolanin K, Mistrik M, et al. Evaluation of candidate biomarkers to predict cancer cell sensitivity or resistance to PARP-1 inhibitor treatment. Cell Cycle. 2012;**11**(20):3837-3850. DOI: 10.4161/cc.22026

[33] Altmeyer M. Addicted to PAR? A closer look at PARP inhibitor sensitivity. Cell Cycle. 2012;**11**(21):3916. DOI: 10.4161/cc.22393

Chapter 6

Genomic Consequences of Ovarian Cancer with Respect to DNA Damage and Repair Mechanism

Sonali Verma, Gresh Chander, Ruchi Shah and Rakesh Kumar

Abstract

Ovarian cancer is not a single disorder having different histological types which are associated with germline or somatic mutations. Histological types include epithelial cancers that account for ~90% of ovarian cancers and include serous, endometrioid, clear-cell and mucinous carcinomas. There are several risk factors for developing ovarian cancer which includes a genetic factor, age, use of hormonal therapy after menopause, null parity, infertility and other factors including obesity, lifestyle, dietary habits. *BRCA1 and BRCA2* are germ line mutations which are completely associated with epithelial ovarian cancer. Germ line mutations in DNA repair pathway which increase the risk of ovarian cancer such as *RAD51C, RAD51D, BRIP1, BARD1, and PALB2*. To understand the mechanism of progression of ovarian cancer it is very important to explore the mechanism behind the abruption of DNA repair genes that are associated with a high risk of ovarian cancer (such as *BRCA1* and *BRCA2*). The study of these DNA repair genes holds a promise for identifying the women at high risk of developing the ovarian cancer in early stages. The main aim of this review is to investigate the development and progression of ovarian cancer and to explore the various genetic and non-genetic perspectives of cancer with special emphasis to personalized medicine.

Keywords: ovarian cancer (OC), high-grade serous carcinoma (HGSC), hormone replacement therapy (HRT), receptor-associated protein 80 (*RAP80)*

1. Introduction

Ovarian cancer is a complex disease with the different biological mechanism at the clinical, cellular and molecular levels. It was clinically proved that ovarian cancer generally presents as a complicated cystic mass in the abdominal region of women. Due to this fact ovarian cancer has been termed the 'mute murderer'; because majority of females have normal symptoms, even when the malignancy is still limited to the ovaries [1].

Majority of ovarian cancer symptoms are still very common where no one knows exactly why some women gets it and others does not. However, same symptoms are shared with many other common gastrointestinal, genitourinary and gynecological disorders and have not yet proved critical for early diagnosis. Ovarian cancer not only starts from ovaries but also originated from other nearby organs like HGSCs start from fallopian tube, peritoneum, endometrial tissue which located outside the uterus known as endometriosis [2]. WHO classifies the Ovarian cancer as tubal cancers [3]. Sometimes knowledge about the primary sites of ovarian cancer has facilitated the prevention strategies for the examination of an advanced stage of ovarian cancer, such as risk reducing and salpingectomy (Surgical removal of fallopian tube) [4]. The aim of this study is to gain a better knowledge of progression of ovarian cancer and how an abruption in DNA repair pathway could predispose one to ovarian cancer, this may help in modification and improvement of drug treatment for developing personalized medicine.

2. Histological types of ovarian carcinoma

The histological types of ovarian cancer can be distinguished into different types which based on risk factors, cells of origin, molecular compositions, clinical features and treatments. These histological types include epithelial cancers that account for ~90% of ovarian cancers and include serous, endometrioid, clear-cell and mucinous carcinomas.

1. High-grade serous carcinoma and high-grade endometrioid carcinoma can present with peritoneal carcinomatosis, ascites and/or pelvic mass or typically advanced stage at presentation in middle aged women (median reported age 50–65 years). These carcinomas are associated with *BRCA* and *TP53* mutations.

2. Low-grade serous carcinoma presents in younger patients (median reported age: 43–55 years) and can be early or late stage at presentation. This type of carcinoma is associated with *KRAS* and *BRAF* mutations and tumors have genomic stability.

3. Low-grade endometrioid carcinoma (median average age of diagnosis-60 years) can be associated with endometriosis and associated with *PTEN, ARID1A* and *PIK3CA* mutations. These mutations have microsatellite instability.

4. Clear-cell carcinoma (median average age of diagnosis-55 years) can present with parenchymal metastases (in the liver and the lungs) and can be associated with hypercoagulability and hypercalcemia which is associated with *ARID1A* and *PIK3CA* mutations

5. Mucinous carcinoma is presents in younger patients (median average age of diagnosis-55 years) and is typically early stage at presentation which associated with *KRAS* mutations [5–7].

3. Incidence and mortality

Every year about, 225,500 new cases of ovarian cancer are diagnosed in all over the world having a death of about 140,200 ovarian cancer patients [8, 9]. Among all of the countries of the world, Russia and UK have the highest rate of ovarian cancer as compared to China is having the lowest rate of ovarian cancer [9]. Annually about 22,280 new cases of ovarian cancer were diagnosed in the US with projected number of deaths for 2016 is 14240 [10, 11]. However, the annual death rate due to ovarian cancer is decreased by 1.09% for women from 1998 to 2008 due to the adoption of new and changing method of hormonal therapy in females [12]. The overall survival rate of ovarian cancer totally depends on the stage of diagnosis; it was reported that the stage 1 patients 92.1% survive for 5 years but is 25% patients with stage III and stage IV cancer [10, 13]. As per 2006 assessment by Indian Council of Medical Research, females (0.428 million) are more susceptible to cancer than males (0.390 million) [14] and ovarian cancer ranks third among all types of cancer in females in India [14]. The rise in the prevalence of ovarian cancer makes it very important to understand the genetic status of cancer among different female population groups of India.

4. Risk factors

There are several risk factors for developing the ovarian cancer which includes genetic factor, age, use of hormonal therapy after menopause, null parity, infertility and other factors including obesity, lifestyle, dietary habits.

4.1 Reproductive factors

Previous studies have described various other factors that can induce the possibility of ovarian cancer, such as parity, prior tubal ligation, salpingectomy and unilateral or bilateral oophorectomy (surgical removal of the ovary) [15]. Even birth giving women have a reduced risk of all subtypes of ovarian cancer compared with women who have not given birth. There is a 30% risk reduction of ovarian cancer in women who undergo treatment of unilateral oophorectomy and bilateral oophorectomy, which is not specific to the particular histological subtype. It was found that women with *BRCA* mutations follow bilateral oophorectomy have 1.1% reduced the risk of ovarian cancer [13, 16]. Other preventive measures to avoid or to reduce the ovarian cancer is tubal ligation, hysterectomy [17]. Some studies have been identified that the breastfeeding and tubal ligation show decreased risk of ovarian cancer in women with germline (*BRCA*) mutation of ovarian cancer [15].

4.2 Hormone replacement therapy

Hormone replacement therapy (*HRT*) has been shown to elevate the possibility of developing ovarian cancer in postmenopausal women; only estrogen therapy promotes the risk by 22% and the both estrogen and progesterone therapy elevate the risk by 10% [18, 19]. Various meta-analysis studies also showed that regular use of hormone replacement therapy either combined progesterone and estrogen or single estrogen elevate the chance of ovarian cancer in menopausal women [20]. It was reported that women having menopausal symptoms and also diagnosed with ovarian cancer the use of hormone replacement therapy appear to be safe and overall has no effect on her survival. Thus it was proved that the hormone replacement therapy can be advised if women having serious menopausal symptoms [21].

5. Other factors

5.1 Obesity

Various previous studies have identified that the obesity is likely to risk factor for ovarian cancer in women. One Meta-analysis studies showed that there is 13%

elevation in risk of ovarian cancer in postmenopausal women with weight gain who did not use any therapy of hormones [22].

5.2 Dietary habits

Several studies have investigated the association between the risk of ovarian cancer and dietary factors in the general population. Milk consumption does not advise any serious risk of ovarian cancer, but some limited studies have recognized a trend that showed a contrary association between the intake of skimmed milk and lactose in adulthood and risk of developing ovarian cancer [23]. Some studies reported that other dietary factors like including vitamins and flavonoids also associate with ovarian cancer [24–26] but it was proven that regular intake of vitamins A, C and E, flavonoids does not cause any ovarian cancer, whereas intake of flavonoids and black tea might be associated with decreased risk of ovarian cancer [27].

5.3 Lifestyle factors

Some other lifestyle factors include the use of talc powder, medications such as NSAIDS and smoking might be a cause of ovarian cancer [28]. Some studies prove that regular use of talcum powder is associated with ovarian cancer but others not [29, 30] Use of aspirin was also associated with decreased risk of developing ovarian cancer, especially among women who took daily, low-dose aspirin, regardless of their age [31]. Cigarette smoking was associated with a significantly lower risk of clear-cell carcinoma but an increased risk of mucinous carcinoma [26].

6. Genetics

The increased risk of ovarian cancer is associated with various genetic factors like *BRCA1, BRCA2, BARD1,BRIPI, RAD51c, RAD51d, PALB2,MSH2,MSH6, MSH1,PMS2* [32, 33]. *BRCA1 and BRCA2* mutations is one of the most predictable genes which are associated with the genetic risk factor of not only ovarian cancer but also with the other cancers in humans (breast, Prostate, melanoma) [34, 35]. Germ line mutations like *BRCA1 and BRCA2* are completely associated with epithelial ovarian cancer but rarely with mucinous ovarian cancer [36]. It was proved that *BRCA2* mutation carrier in ovarian cancer kill more cancer cells and survive more as compared to wild type because *BRCA2* carrier is strongly associated with increased sensitivity to platinum [36, 37]. Both *BRCA* loci strongly associated with both breast and ovarian cancer. There are also genetic germ line mutations in DNA repair pathway which increase the risk of ovarian cancer such as *RAD51C, RAD51D, BRIP1, BARD1 and PALB2* [33, 38, 39]. Other inherited mutations of DNA repair pathway which are strongly associated with ovarian cancer are *CHEK2, MRE11A, RAD50, ATM* and *TP53* [33, 35, 38]. One major cause of ovarian cancer is Lynch syndrome as it is also associated with colorectal, endometrial urinary tract, stomach, small intestine and biliary tract cancers. Lynch syndrome is a mark of germ line mutation in genes *MLH1, PMS2, MSH2 or MSH6*, of DNA mismatch repair system [40, 41]. The specific reasons why these inherited mutated genes are involved in specific organs are not known yet.

The most commonly studied genetic alterations in ovarian cancer are those which involved in DNA repair. The mutations of both somatic or germline in homologous recombination genes have been recognized in nearly one- third one-third of ovarian carcinomas, comprising of both serous and non-serous histological types and subtypes that were not formerly admitted to having characteristics of homologous recombination deficiency (clear-cell and endometrioid carcinomas, as well as carcinosarcoma) [42]. As previously discussed, the frequently involved inherited genes are *BRCA1, BRCA2, and BRIP1*, genes that are part of the Fanconi anemia pathway (*RAD51C, RAD51D, BRIP1, PALB2 and BARD1*) and genes that are involved in DNA mismatch repair (*MSH2, MSH6, MLH1 and PMS2)* [43]. Although genomic data exhibit recurrent mutations in patients with ovarian cancer, some tumors, specifically the HGSC subtype, are genetically heterogeneous [43, 44] following the basic genomic complexity of this disease.

TP53 is driver mutation and ubiquitous in high-grade ovarian carcinoma. *TP53* is the utmost mutated gene in HGSC [43]. *TP53* commonly occur in the encoding region of the gene i.e., in DNA Binding domain and non-DNA binding domains. *TP53* mutations can be missense or nonsense, frameshift insertions and deletions [45]. Lack of *TP53* mutations in tumors have p53 Dys-functioning with a gain of copy number of *MDM2* or *MDM4*, These *MDM2* or *MDM4* involved in regulation and degradation of *P53* [45]. Some former studies of Genomic examination have disclosed the imperfections in homologous recombination in ~50% of analyzed HGSCs [34]. Imperfective homologous recombination is correlated with both germline and somatic *BRCA* mutations, as well as modifications in other DNA repair pathway genes [46]. The properties of *BRCA1* is critical for DNA repair, cell cycle checkpoint control, mitosis, remodeling of chromatin and transcriptional regulation; whereas *BRCA2* is important in homologous recombination and DNA repair [47].

Most common recurrent molecular modifications analyzed in ovarian carcinoma especially in high-grade serous carcinoma are defective Notch, phosphoinositide 3-kinases (*PI3K), RAS–MEK* and fork head box protein M1 (*FOXM1*) signaling pathways, there is a change in somatic copy number in the genes which encode proteins of these signaling pathways [46]. Some genes (*AURKA, ERBB3, CDK2, mTOR, BRD4, and MYC*) after mutation play an important role in the pathogenesis of ovarian carcinoma (High- grade serous carcinoma) and also act as therapeutic agents for ovarian cancer [48, 49].

Generally, ovarian cancer shares a common origin within ovarian surface epithelium (OSE). During the process of monthly ovulation in the female reproductive system, the OSE is degraded enzymatically in order to admit the follicular rupture and releasing of oocyte which creates a gap that must be repaired [50]. Throughout the period of a woman's reproductive life, the process of damage and repair is continuously repeated many times will result in a bit by bit aggregation of genomic alterations, as hypothesized by the continuous ovulation hypothesis [51]. In inclusion of physical trauma, ovarian surface cells are subjected to ovulation-associated inflammatory cytokines, reactive oxygen species (ROS), and hormones (and its reactive metabolites) that are able to damage DNA and lead to an imbalance of hormonal metabolism [52]. In ovaries, cysts develop as an ovulation occur due to aging or becoming entrapped within the stroma. When cysts left with DNA damage, they may be the best spot for the progression of malignancy [53]. The association between DNA damage and ovarian cancer becomes stronger, so it will become important to thoroughly understand the role of DNA damage response (DDR) proteins in Ovarian cancer prevention. The identification of DNA damage and their resultant repair mechanism are critical in perspective of response or resistance of cancer cells to treatment. This means that cells with their particular DNA damage repair pathways are able to effectively repair the damage caused by chemo or radiotherapy, being responsible for the improvement of resistance in tumor cells [54, 55].

7. DNA damage and repair

In ovarian cancer, the process of DNA damage of double stranded DNA and homologous repair (shown in **Figure 1**) starts with identification of double-strand breaks (DSBs) by the process of meiotic recombination 11 homolog 1 (*MRE11)–RAD50*–Nijmegen breakage syndrome protein 1 (*NBS1) (MRN*) complex, both

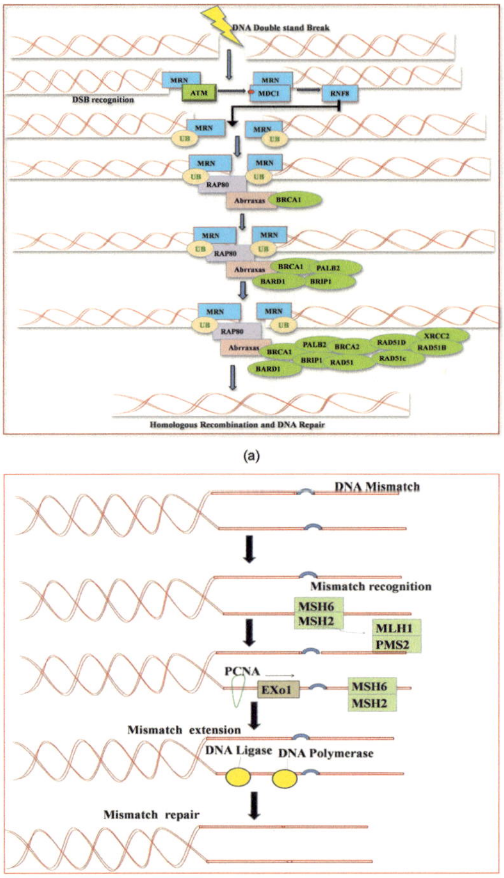

Figure 1.

Double strand DNA damage and homologous repair: When DNA damage with any external agent takes place, ATM (ataxia telangiectasia mutated) act as main part of homologous recombination, it phosphorylates H2AX (histone family member X). ATM compliment and attach with mediator of DNA damage checkpoint protein 1 (MDC1) and NBS1 (Nijmegen breakage syndrome 1) of the MRN complex. The binding site for binding site for the E3 ubiquitin-protein ligase RING finger protein 8 (RNF8) is created after phosphorylation of MDC1. The phosphorylation leads to mediate the organization of downstream proteins involved with DNA damage response such as receptor-associated protein 80 (RAP80; encoded by UIMC1). For the interaction of BRCA1 breast cancer type 1 susceptibility protein (BRCA1) with RAP80 for the repair of DNA break, the abraxas (encoded by FAM175A) act as mediator adaptor protein. BRCA1-associated RING domain protein 1 (BARD1) and BRCA1-interacting protein 1 (BRIP1; also known as Fanconi anemia group J protein) forms heterodimer. BRCA lift other DNA repair protein like RAD51 (DNA repair homology), XRCC1 (X-ray repair cross complementing 1), BRIP1 proteins which helps in the repair of DNA break. Mismatch repair: In the process of DNA mismatch the PMS2 (PMS1 homolog 2, mismatch repair system component) & MSH (MutS protein homolog 2) as a main initiator which helps in the proliferation of cell nuclear antigen. The abnormalities in any MUTl protein homolog led to mismatch in DNA repair. This mismatch is further harnessing the exonuclease 1 (EXO) for the removal of mismatch for the correction of double strand break with ligase and polymerase activity.

(MRE11)–RAD50 act as a stimulation site for the serine-protein kinase ATM. In DNA repair pathway, *ATM* plays an important role with a combination of homologous recombination. The phosphorylation of histone *H2AX* by *ATM* which ultimately attach with the mediator of DNA damage checkpoint protein 1 (*MDC1*) and *NBS1* of the *MRN* complex for the enhancement of *ATM* binding. The phosphorylation of *MDC1* helps in the formation of the binding site for the E3 ubiquitin-protein ligase RING finger protein 8 (*RNF8*), This admits ubiquitin-mediated enlistment of downstream DNA damage response proteins, such as receptor-associated protein 80 (*RAP80*; encoded by *UIMC1*), Whereas *RAP80* is an important ubiquitin-interaction motif-containing protein that accomplice with the breast cancer type 1 susceptibility protein (*BRCA1*) complex over its communication with Abraxas (encoded by *FAM175A*); The main function of Abraxas is acting as middle adaptor protein and contains domains essential for *BRCA1* interactions [46]. The *RAP80*–Abraxas compositely is critical for placing *BRCA1* to the site of DNA repair. Both *BRCA1* and *BRCA2* act as scaffolds for other types of proteins involved in DNA repair. *BRCA1*-associated RING domain protein 1 (*BARD1*) and *BRCA1*-interacting protein 1 (*BRIP1*; also known as Fanconi anemia group J protein) attach precisely to *BRCA1*; whereas *BARD1* in collaboration with *BRCA1* forms a heterodimer which is most important for collective stability [42]. In addition, *BRIP1* also attach to *BRCA1* which is important and compulsory for activation of check-point of S phase. Companion and localizer of *BRCA2 (PALB2)* help *BRCA1 and BRCA2* attach at sites of DNA damage and helps to lift the *RAD51* proteins on to the *BRCA* proteins; the DNA repair protein *XRCC2* is one of the five forewords of *RAD51*. When genes of homologous repair get mutated it will lead to accumulation of various double strands break So due to this way there is a formation of defective DNA repair pathway and in future, this will increase the chance of developing ovarian cancer [42].

7.1 Mismatch repair

DNA Mismatch repair (MMR) corrects single base impairs as it identifies and repairs false insertion, deletion and mis-incorporation of nucleotides [56]. DNA mismatch repair pathway (Shown in is started by the *MutS* protein homolog 2 (*MSH*) proteins, as well as the endonuclease *PMS2* which proliferate cell nuclear antigen (*PCNA*). In ovarian cancer, the mutation in genes encoding *MutL* protein homolog 1 *(MLH1), MSH2, MSH6* and *PMS2* there is an abnormality in DNA mismatch repair pathway [56]. Attachment of this complex to the mismatched bases facilitates the recruitment of *MLH1* and *PMS2*. *PCNA* bind to the sites of base mismatch and assist to recruit and harness exonuclease 1 (*EXO1*; a member of the *RAD2* exonuclease family) to the place of DNA damage. *EXO1* excises the mismatched bases, which are then corrected by DNA polymerase and DNA ligase [42].

BRCA1 and *BRCA2* are key genes which play important role DNA repair where *BRCA1*-associated RING domain protein 1 (*BARD1*) forms stable heterodimers with *BRCA1* and this communication is important for the action of *BRCA1* [57]. Therefore *BARD1* improve efficient Homologous repair [58]. Collaborator and localizer of *BRCA2 (PALB2)* collaborate with both *BRCA1* and *BRCA2*, and functions downstream of *BRCA1*, as the corporation with *BRCA1* promote recruitment of *PALB2* to damaged DNA [59]. *PALB2* also combine directly with and maintain *BRCA2* during the creation of the *RAD51* nucleoprotein filament [60]. *ATM* then phosphorylates *PALB2* to help *RAD51* nucleoprotein filament maintenance [61]. Current data advise that the *BRCA1– PALB2* interaction is regulated by the cell cycle to restrain homologous recombination repair in G1 phase, where the sister chromatid is not applicable for Homologous repair. This regulatory step regulates false by reducing the use of the homologous chromosome for homologous repair or the direct annealing of resected ends, which possibly could lead to loss of resected DNA pieces [62]. The *RAD51* prefaces (*RAD51B, RAD51C, RAD51D, XRCC2*, and *XRCC3*) are also critical for *RAD51* nucleoprotein filament formation, even though their exact mechanism is still unknown [63]. Some previous studies reported that the pathogenic mutations in *BARD1* and *PALB2* are significantly associated with an increased risk of breast cancer [64–66], when in fact the lifetime risk for ovarian cancer is suggested to be low [67]. It was reported in two studies that deleterious *RAD51B* mutations in patients with breast or ovarian cancer, but no risk estimates are currently available [68, 69]. In spite of recent report of pathogenic *RAD51C* mutations, truncating mutations in *RAD51C* and *RAD51D* are found mainly in families with ovarian cancer only or breast and ovarian cancer [70]. Rare mutations in *XRCC2* have been advised to increase the risk of breast and ovarian cancer [71] but the data were not proved by another report [72]; therefore, large number studies are essential before *XRCC2* can be regarded as an important Hereditary Breast and Ovarian Cancer gene. *BRCA1*-interacting protein carboxy-terminal helicase 1 (*BRIP1*; also known as Fanconi anemia group J protein (*FANCJ*)) and *BRCA1-A* complex subunit Abraxas (encoded by *FAM175A*) are also recommended to be involved in homologous repair by recruiting BRCA1 to DSBs [39]. The *BRIP1* gene was basically advised to be a low-penetrant breast cancer susceptibility gene [73]. Easton et al., 2016 in their study proved that *BRIP1* gene is not associated with an augmented risk of breast and ovarian cancer [74]. However, in some studies it was proved that carriers of *BRIP1* mutation have a high risk for ovarian cancer [75]. There are various Pathogenic mutations have been identified in patients with ovarian cancer [76, 77], but the lifetime risk of ovarian cancer is still unknown.

8. Summary and future perspective of study

In ovarian cancer, the status of molecular alterations especially at the time of diagnosis is change over time due to the presence of some few driver mutations (*XRCC1, RAD51*) which is based on platinum-based drugs or due to the presence of large number of changes in copy number of genes of various signaling pathways which always characterize the complexity of genome of ovarian cancer.

Actually, this molecular complication support insight into perhaps why the advancement of effective therapies for ovarian carcinoma (especially high-grade serous carcinoma) has been problematic to attain. Various recent literature has shown the role of various DNA damage and repair signaling pathways in ovarian cancer in the world. However, such studies are lacking in Indian population. Studying the role of coding and noncoding genes in ovarian cancer pathogenesis will add to our understanding of the genetic landscape of ovarian cancer and our study may highlight the novel pathway associated with the disease other than the conventional pathways. Associated coding and noncoding genes can be targeted for development of new therapeutic strategies and a new step towards personalized medicine.

Author details

Sonali Verma[1*], Gresh Chander[1], Ruchi Shah[2] and Rakesh Kumar[1*]

1 Indian Council of Medical Research-Centre for Advance Research, Shri Mata Vaishno Devi University, Katra, J&K, India

2 Department of Biotechnology, Kashmir University, J&K, India

*Address all correspondence to: Sonali.verma@smvdu.ac.in
and kumar.rakesh@smvdu.ac.in

References

[1] Goff BA et al. Ovarian carcinoma diagnosis. Cancer. 2000;**89**(10): 2068-2075

[2] Pentheroudakis G, Pavlidis N. Serous papillary peritoneal carcinoma: Unknown primary tumour, ovarian cancer counterpart or a distinct entity? A systematic review. Critical Reviews in Oncology/Hematology. 2010;**75**(1):27-42

[3] Cree IA, White VA, Indave BI Lokuhetty D. Revising the WHO classification: Female genital tract tumours. Histopathology. 2020;**76**:151-156. DOI: 10.1111/his.13977

[4] Kindelberger DW et al. Intraepithelial carcinoma of the fimbria and pelvic serous carcinoma: Evidence for a causal relationship. The American Journal of Surgical Pathology. 2007;**31**(2):161-169

[5] Groen RS, Gershenson DM, Fader AN. Updates and emerging therapies for rare epithelial ovarian cancers: One size no longer fits all. Gynecologic Oncology. 2015;**136**(2):373-383

[6] Mangili G et al. Unraveling the two entities of endometrioid ovarian cancer: A single center clinical experience. Gynecologic Oncology. 2012;**126**(3):403-407

[7] Oswald AJ, Gourley C. Low-grade epithelial ovarian cancer: A number of distinct clinical entities? Current Opinion in Oncology. 2015;**27**(5):412-419

[8] Lowe KA et al. An international assessment of ovarian cancer incidence and mortality. Gynecologic Oncology. 2013;**130**(1):107-114

[9] Sung P-L et al. Global distribution pattern of histological subtypes of epithelial ovarian cancer: A database analysis and systematic review. Gynecologic Oncology. 2014;**133**(2):147-154

[10] Siegel RL, Miller KD, Jemal A. Cancer statistics, 2016. CA: a Cancer Journal for Clinicians. 2016;**66**(1):7-30

[11] Siegel RL, Miller KD, Jemal A. Cancer statistics, 2017. CA: a Cancer Journal for Clinicians. 2017;**67**(1):7-30

[12] Yang HP et al. Ovarian cancer incidence trends in relation to changing patterns of menopausal hormone therapy use in the United States. Journal of Clinical Oncology. 2013;**31**(17):2146-2151

[13] Rice MS, Hankinson SE, Tworoger SS. Tubal ligation, hysterectomy, unilateral oophorectomy, and risk of ovarian cancer in the nurses' health studies. Fertility and Sterility. 2014;**102**(1):192-198. e3

[14] D'Souza ND, Murthy N, Aras R. Projection of cancer incident cases for India-till 2026. Asian Pacific Journal of Cancer Prevention. 2013;**14**(7):4379-4386

[15] Friebel TM, Domchek SM, Rebbeck TR. Modifiers of cancer risk in BRCA1 and BRCA2 mutation carriers: A systematic review and meta-analysis. JNCI: Journal of the National Cancer Institute. 2014;**106**(6)

[16] Domchek SM et al. Association of risk-reducing surgery in BRCA1 or BRCA2 mutation carriers with cancer risk and mortality. JAMA. 2010;**304**(9):967-975

[17] Gaitskell K et al. Tubal ligation and ovarian cancer risk in a large cohort:

Substantial variation by histological type. International Journal of Cancer. 2016;**138**(5):1076-1084

[18] Pearce CL et al. Increased ovarian cancer risk associated with menopausal estrogen therapy is reduced by adding a progestin. Cancer. 2009;**115**(3):531-539

[19] Hildebrand JS et al. Postmenopausal hormone use and incident ovarian cancer: Associations differ by regimen. International Journal of Cancer. 2010;**127**(12):2928-2935

[20] Cancer, C.G.o.E.S.o.O. Menopausal hormone use and ovarian cancer risk: Individual participant meta-analysis of 52 epidemiological studies. The Lancet. 2015;**385**(9980):1835-1842

[21] Eeles RA et al. Adjuvant hormone therapy may improve survival in epithelial ovarian cancer: Results of the AHT randomized trial. Journal of Clinical Oncology. 2015;**33**(35):4138-4144

[22] Keum N et al. Adult weight gain and adiposity-related cancers: A dose-response meta-analysis of prospective observational studies. Journal of the National Cancer Institute. 2015;**107**(2):djv088

[23] Merritt MA et al. Dairy food and nutrient intake in different life periods in relation to risk of ovarian cancer. Cancer Causes & Control. 2014;**25**(7):795-808

[24] Koushik A et al. Intake of vitamins a, C, and E and folate and the risk of ovarian cancer in a pooled analysis of 10 cohort studies. Cancer Causes & Control. 2015;**26**(9):1315-1327

[25] Xie J et al. A prospective cohort study of dietary indices and incidence of epithelial ovarian cancer. Journal of Ovarian Research. 2014;7(1):112

[26] Wentzensen N et al. Ovarian cancer risk factors by histologic subtype: An analysis from the ovarian cancer cohort consortium. Journal of Clinical Oncology. 2016;**34**(24):2888-2898

[27] Cassidy A et al. Intake of dietary flavonoids and risk of epithelial ovarian cancer. The American Journal of Clinical Nutrition. 2014:ajcn. 088708

[28] Cramer DW et al. The association between talc use and ovarian cancer: A retrospective case–control study in two US states. Epidemiology (Cambridge, Mass.). 2016;**27**(3):334

[29] Terry KL et al. Genital powder use and risk of ovarian cancer: A pooled analysis of 8,525 cases and 9,859 controls. Cancer Prevention Research. 2013:canprevres. 0037.2013

[30] Houghton SC et al. Perineal powder use and risk of ovarian cancer. JNCI: Journal of the National Cancer Institute. 2014;**106**(9)

[31] Trabert B et al. Aspirin, nonaspirin nonsteroidal anti-inflammatory drug, and acetaminophen use and risk of invasive epithelial ovarian cancer: A pooled analysis in the ovarian cancer association consortium. JNCI: Journal of the National Cancer Institute. 2014;**106**(2)

[32] Zhang S et al. Frequencies of BRCA1 and BRCA2 mutations among 1,342 unselected patients with invasive ovarian cancer. Gynecologic Oncology. 2011;**121**(2):353-357

[33] Norquist BM et al. Inherited mutations in women with ovarian carcinoma. JAMA Oncology. 2016;**2**(4):482-490

[34] Alsop K et al. BRCA mutation frequency and patterns of treatment

response in BRCA mutation–positive women with ovarian cancer: A report from the Australian ovarian cancer study group. Journal of Clinical Oncology. 2012;**30**(21):2654-2663

[35] Pennington KP, Swisher EM. Hereditary ovarian cancer: Beyond the usual suspects. Gynecologic Oncology. 2012;**124**(2):347-353

[36] Bolton KL et al. Association between BRCA1 and BRCA2 mutations and survival in women with invasive epithelial ovarian cancer. JAMA. 2012;**307**(4):382-389

[37] Liu G et al. Differing clinical impact of BRCA1 and BRCA2 mutations in serous ovarian cancer. Pharmacogenomics. 2012;**13**(13):1523-1535

[38] Walsh T et al. Mutations in 12 genes for inherited ovarian, fallopian tube, and peritoneal carcinoma identified by massively parallel sequencing. Proceedings of the National Academy of Sciences. 2011;**108**(44):18032-18037

[39] Prakash R et al. Homologous recombination and human health: The roles of BRCA1, BRCA2, and associated proteins. Cold Spring Harbor Perspectives in Biology. 2015;**7**(4):a016600

[40] Ketabi Z et al. Ovarian cancer linked to lynch syndrome typically presents as early-onset, non-serous epithelial tumors. Gynecologic Oncology. 2011;**121**(3):462-465

[41] Engel C et al. Risks of less common cancers in proven mutation carriers with lynch syndrome. Journal of Clinical Oncology. 2012;**30**(35):4409-4415

[42] Matulonis UA et al. Ovarian Cancer. 2016;**2**:16061

[43] Patch A-M et al. Whole-genome characterization of chemoresistant ovarian cancer. Nature. 2015;**521**(7553):489

[44] Bashashati A et al. Distinct evolutionary trajectories of primary high-grade serous ovarian cancers revealed through spatial mutational profiling. The Journal of Pathology. 2013;**231**(1):21-34

[45] Ahmed AA et al. Driver mutations in TP53 are ubiquitous in high grade serous carcinoma of the ovary. The Journal of Pathology. 2010;**221**(1):49-56

[46] Network CGAR. Integrated genomic analyses of ovarian carcinoma. Nature. 2011;**474**(7353):609

[47] O'donovan PJ, Livingston DM. BRCA1 and BRCA2: Breast/ovarian cancer susceptibility gene products and participants in DNA double-strand break repair. Carcinogenesis. 2010;**31**(6):961-967

[48] Baratta MG et al. An in-tumor genetic screen reveals that the BET bromodomain protein, BRD4, is a potential therapeutic target in ovarian carcinoma. Proceedings of the National Academy of Sciences. 2015;**112**(1):232-237

[49] Reyes-González JM et al. Targeting c-MYC in platinum-resistant ovarian cancer. Molecular Cancer Therapeutics. 2015;**14**(10):2260-2269

[50] Murdoch WJ, McDonnel AC. Roles of the ovarian surface epithelium in ovulation and carcinogenesis. Reproduction. 2002;**123**(6):743-750

[51] Fathalla MF. Incessant ovulation—A factor in ovarian neoplasia? The Lancet. 1971;**298**(7716):163

[52] Ness RB, Cottreau C. Possible role of ovarian epithelial inflammation in ovarian cancer. Journal of the National Cancer Institute. 1999;**91**(17):1459-1467

[53] Karst AM, Drapkin R. Ovarian cancer pathogenesis: A model in evolution. Journal of Oncology. 2009;**2010**

[54] Christmann M et al. Mechanisms of human DNA repair: An update. Toxicology. 2003;**193**(1):3-34

[55] Assis J, Pereira D, Medeiros R. Ovarian cancer and DNA repair: DNA ligase IV as a potential key. World Journal of Clinical Oncology. 2013;**4**(1):14

[56] Nielsen FC, van Overeem Hansen T, Sørensen CS. Hereditary breast and ovarian cancer: New genes in confined pathways. Nature Reviews Cancer. 2016;**16**(9):599-612

[57] Shakya R et al. The basal-like mammary carcinomas induced by Brca1 or Bard1 inactivation implicate the BRCA1/BARD1 heterodimer in tumor suppression. Proceedings of the National Academy of Sciences. 2008;**105**(19):7040-7045

[58] Lee C et al. Functional analysis of BARD1 missense variants in homology-directed repair of DNA double Strand breaks. Human Mutation. 2015;**36**(12):1205-1214

[59] Zhang F et al. PALB2 links BRCA1 and BRCA2 in the DNA-damage response. Current Biology. 2009;**19**(6):524-529

[60] Buisson R et al. Cooperation of breast cancer proteins PALB2 and piccolo BRCA2 in stimulating homologous recombination. Nature Structural & Molecular Biology. 2010;**17**(10):1247-1254

[61] Ahlskog JK et al. ATM/ATR-mediated phosphorylation of PALB2 promotes RAD51 function. EMBO Reports. 2016;**17**(5):671-681

[62] Orthwein A et al. A mechanism for the suppression of homologous recombination in G1 cells. Nature. 2015;**528**(7582):422

[63] Suwaki N, Klare K, Tarsounas M. RAD51 paralogs: Roles in DNA damage signalling, recombinational repair and tumorigenesis. In: Seminars in Cell & Developmental Biology. Elsevier; 2011

[64] De Brakeleer S et al. Cancer predisposing missense and protein truncating BARD1 mutations in non-BRCA1 or BRCA2 breast cancer families. Human Mutation. 2010;**31**(3)

[65] Rahman N et al. PALB2, which encodes a BRCA2-interacting protein, is a breast cancer susceptibility gene. Nature Genetics. 2007;**39**(2):165

[66] Erkko H et al. A recurrent mutation in PALB2 in Finnish cancer families. Nature. 2007;**446**(7133):316

[67] Ramus SJ et al. Germline mutations in the BRIP1, BARD1, PALB2, and NBN genes in women with ovarian cancer. JNCI: Journal of the National Cancer Institute. 2015;**107**(11)

[68] Golmard L et al. Germline mutation in the RAD51B gene confers predisposition to breast cancer. BMC Cancer. 2013;**13**(1):484

[69] Song H et al. Contribution of germline mutations in the RAD51B, RAD51C, and RAD51D genes to ovarian cancer in the population. Journal of Clinical Oncology. 2015;**33**(26):2901-2907

[70] Loveday C et al. Germline mutations in RAD51D confer susceptibility to ovarian cancer. Nature Genetics. 2011;**43**(9):879-882

[71] Park D et al. Rare mutations in XRCC2 increase the risk of breast cancer. The American Journal of Human Genetics. 2012;**90**(4):734-739

[72] Hilbers FS et al. Rare variants in XRCC2 as breast cancer susceptibility alleles. Journal of Medical Genetics. 2012;**49**(10):618-620

[73] Seal S et al. Truncating mutations in the Fanconi anemia J gene BRIP1 are low-penetrance breast cancer susceptibility alleles. Nature Genetics. 2006;**38**(11):1239

[74] Easton DF et al. No evidence that protein truncating variants in BRIP1 are associated with breast cancer risk: Implications for gene panel testing. Journal of Medical Genetics. 2016;**53**(5):298-309

[75] Rafnar T et al. Mutations in BRIP1 confer high risk of ovarian cancer. Nature Genetics. 2011;**43**(11):1104-1107

[76] Solyom S et al. Breast cancer–associated abraxas mutation disrupts nuclear localization and DNA damage response functions. Science Translational Medicine. 2012;**4**(122):122ra23 122ra23

[77] Pennington KP et al. Germline and somatic mutations in homologous recombination genes predict platinum response and survival in ovarian, fallopian tube, and peritoneal carcinomas. Clinical Cancer Research. 2014;**20**(3):764-775

Section 5

BRCA Genetic Testing and Counselling

Chapter 7

Implications of BRCA1 and BRCA2 Mutations in Mexico

Carlos Arturo Gonzalez Nuñez, Paula Anel Cabrera Galeana, Sandy Ruiz Cruz and Alexandra Garcilazo Reyes

Abstract

BRCA 1 or BRCA 2 mutations have played a role in understanding its risk for several different cancer like breast, ovarian, prostate, and pancreatic cancer Knowing that biology is king, and its determination plays a role in prognosis for patients with cancer. Several recommendations have been made focusing on which population should have BRCA mutational status determined. This determination could help seek targeted therapy that could have a beneficial impact on cancer patients. Having this said, efforts have been made to determine if our Mexican population has the same prognosis when BRCA mutation is present when compared to global reports. As well as researching founder mutations that could help understand our Mexican population. This chapter seeks to describe and analysis this current scenario in Mexican population with BRCA mutation.

Keywords: BRCA1, BRCA2, BRCA 1/2, breast cancer, ovarian cancer, prostate cancer, Latin cancer patients, Mexican cancer patients, Mexico, founder mutations

1. Introduction

BRCA 1 or BRCA 2 mutations, implicate a different prognosis depending on the type of neoplasm its associated with. Having this said, in ovarian cancer, those with BRCA mutational status have been associated with a better prognosis compared to those without BRCA mutational status [1]. This also seems to be the case in breast cancer, although different reports have concluded mixed results in the scene that BRCA mutational is not always associated with a better cancer prognosis [2, 3]. These mixed results could probably be explained by different factors, taking in account race, country of origin which could represent different founder BRCA mutations. We would like to describe the prevalence of BRCA 1/2 in Mexico, as well as founder mutations of BRCA in our population, and the impact it translates in our daily practice.

2. BRCA 1/2 mutations and breast cancer in Mexico

Breast cancer is the most common neoplasm worldwide, this also seems to be the case in Mexico; with 195,499 new cases of cancer reported in 2020 of which 15.3%

IntechOpen

(29,929) where associated with breast cancer [4]. Breast cancer has incremented in its incidence and mortality in Mexico during the last three decades, according to the last report made by the Epidemiology Department in the Secretary of Health, with an initial incidence of 10.76 cases per 100,000 habitants to 26.1 cases per 100,000 habitants in women of 25 years of age or older [5]. This clearly depicts how breast cancer is considered a public health problem that requires a focused diagnosis with an accurate treatment, considering the different epidemiology set in our country.

Although breast cancer is the most common cancer, as is mostly reported in the rest of the world there a few differences to consider. In Mexico, the mean age of diagnosis is 52.5 years, considered 10 years younger when compared to the rest of the world. Of these patients, approximately 13.3% are 40 years of age or younger at time of diagnosis [6, 7].

The associations between risk factors and breast cancer in the Latin American population have been considered complex due to the extensive diversity of cultures and ancestral origins that may be contributing for the risk of breast cancer [8].

Mexico has had a demographic, epidemiological and economic transition that has favored the increase of risk factors for breast cancer (increased age, obesity and diabetes) [9]. This younger population should be considered relevant since screening for BRCA 1 or BRCA 2 mutation is recommended for patients younger than 45 years of age with a family history of breast cancer [10].

Some international recommendations for searching for BRCA mutations vary according to associations and regions. For example The National Comprehesive Cancer Network (NCCN) recommends testing in: diagnosis of breast cancer in a patient under 45 years of age, patient between 45 and 50 years of age with synchronous or metachronous breast cancer or associated with a first-degree relative with ovarian, breast, prostate, pancreas, and breast cancer older than 51 years with ovarian cancer, pancreas and finally patient of any age with: triple negative breast cancer, male breast cancer and in which the result can define the use of a PARP inhibitor. The European Society for Medical Oncology (ESMO) recommends BRCA determination in patients with breast cancer if the age upon diagnosis is 40 years or less, as well as those with bilateral breast cancer at the age of 50 or less, and in those with triple negative breast cancer at the age of 60 or less. Two first degree relatives with breast cancer, ovarian cancer, prostate cancer, pancreatic cancer is also motive for BRCA mutational status determination [11].

These screening recommendations are also following in our clinical practice, because there aren't current guidelines in Mexico for the determination of mutation in BRCA 1 and/or BRCA2 extrapolating international guideline recommendations in our daily practice.

Although much of our daily practice is extrapolated from international guidelines. BRCA 1/2 mutations have been a source of investigation for the past decade. In Mexico a prevalence of varying from 17.4 to 30% of BRCA 1 or 2 mutations has been described, [12, 13] which is higher than what has been reported in our countries with 3% in all patients diagnosed with breast cancer, and 20% in those with high-risk families [14]. We previously mentioned that breast cancer is diagnosed at a younger age in Mexico, this could partially explain why prevalence in BRCA mutations is different from what has been described in other countries. Not only is our prevalence different, but also the subtype of breast cancer associated with BRCA mutations. In general, Basal-like subtype breast cancer is associated with BRCA 1 mutation and BRCA 2 with Luminal B-like subtype [15]. In Latin America, 37.1% with BRCA mutations have positive Estrogen and Progesterone receptors, with only 17.8% considered

Triple negative with BRCA mutation, although this was not analyzed according to the type of BRCA mutation [13]. This proves that breast cancer is an heterogenous disease that also differs between countries. This led to an effort in investigating the presence of founder BRCA mutations in Mexico. The Hispanic mutation panel (HISPANEL) was designed due to the need of an inexpensive accessible screening tool to properly diagnosis patients with high for BRCA mutations.

HISPANEL incorporates 115 BRCA mutations observed in Hispanic women. It is estimated that among Mexican women with breast or ovarian cancer it has a sensitivity of 68% [14]. This panel led to the discovery of the first Mexican BRCA founder mutation, BRCA1 ex9–12del large rearrangement, which is present in 12% of all BRCA1 mutations in patients with family history of breast cancer [16].

This was further studied in patients without family history of breast cancer, where 67% patients with locally advanced breast cancer and only 2% with metastatic disease were analyzed [17]. This should be considered an important subjective of discussion due to adjuvant treatment in locally advanced breast cancer as well as second line treatment for metastasis breast cancer with Olaparib [18]. This will further be described in the treatment section. Surprisingly, out of 96 patients with breast cancer analyzed, 29% patients had BRCA1 ex9–12del founder mutation [17].

Some recurrent mutations found in the Mexican population are shown in **Table 1** [19].

This leads us to think that BRCA mutation should be determined in patients with 50 years of age or younger and breast cancer diagnosis, independent of family history for breast cancer. BRCA1 ex9–12del mutation is not routinely analyzed when searching for BRCA mutations in breast cancer patients. An important aspect to consider when determining BRCA mutations is the presence of copy-number variants (CNV), which are hypothesized to have a better prognosis since they are less susceptible to reversal mutations leading to less resistance to DNA-damaging therapies [20]. This was shown in a cohort study from the HISPANEL population, where those patients with BRCA CNV had better overall survival (OS) when compared to those with BRCA pathologic variants at 10 years; respectively 100% vs. 78.6% [13]. The growing access to diagnostic tests for BRCA mutational status could help analyze this information at a larger scale. What is true is due to recent approbation by the Federal Commission for the Protection Against Sanitary Risks (COFEPRIS) for the use of a PARP inhibitor name Olaparib, there has been collaborations with different laboratories in performing a BRCA mutational status test across the country. This has allowed to further indicate PARP inhibitors as a 2nd line treatment option in triple negative metastatic breast cancer, as well as an in hormonal receptor positive HER2 negative metastatic breast cancer, according to NCCN guidelines [18].

Olaparib, a PARP inhibitor, is also used for triple negative early disease breast cancer with residual disease after neoadjuvant chemotherapy, and those with tumor size of 2 cm or axillary node-positive disease who received standard adjuvant

BRCA1 Variant	BRCA2
Ex9–12del	3492insT
185delAG	E49X
R71G	G2793R
R1443X	

Table 1.
BRCA mutations found in Mexican patients.

chemotherapy. In the case of hormone receptor positive HER2 negative early breast cancer, those who received standard adjuvant chemotherapy, who had 4 pathologically confirmed positive lymph nodes or those who received neoadjuvant chemotherapy with a CPS + EG score of 3 or more, should receive Olaparib; considering these scenarios only in those the germline BRCA mutations [21].

For patients with somatic BRCA mutations, there is only information in metastatic breast cancer, which was analyzed in a Phase II clinical trial, observing an objective response of 50%, for those with BRCA somatic mutations [22]. This is an important aspect to consider when determining BRCA mutational status in our patients, considering that most of the information, and approval for certain drugs are in BRCA germline mutations. The difference of at least objective response between germline mutations and somatic BRCA mutations when using PARP inhibitors, like Olaparib, has not been studied in Mexican population with breast cancer. This could be an area of clinical investigation in our field, considering higher access to BRCA mutational determination tests in certain parts of the country.

Another aspect to consider is the sequence of treatment in when to initiate PARP inhibitors in metastatic breast cancer. Most guidelines (ESMO, NCCN) recommend initiating after progressive disease to first line palliative therapy [18, 23]. This could seem straightforward, due to the fact the Olaparib and Talazoparib are not associated with overall survival benefit [24, 25] considering that other first line palliative options are associated with this oncologic outcome (overall survival). This should be considered with caution, considering BRCA germline patients have a different biologic behavior. To set an example, although there is no doubt the CDK4/6 inhibitors combined with hormonal therapy revolutionized different oncologic outcomes in hormone receptor positive HER2 negative metastatic breast cancer, this does not seem to be the case in patients with germline BRCA mutational status. Overall survival is lower in patients with gBRCA mutational status patients who were treated with CDK4/6 inhibitors when compared to those with wild type BRCA mutational status [26], considering this information. It could also be a field of opportunity in investigation frontline CDK 4/6 inhibitors with hormonal therapy versus PARP inhibitors, not only in our Mexican population, but also in other countries. The same question could be asked for HER2 positive patients, where PARP inhibition with antiHER2 therapy has been shown to enhance the effect of antiHER2 therapy like trastuzumab [27].

3. BRCA 1/2 mutations and ovarian cancer in Mexico

Ovarian cancer represents the 14th most common cancer in Mexico, according to GLOBOCAN 2020, ranking itself in 12th place for mortality [4]. This risk could be increased for those with BRCA mutations, from 1.2% to 39–44% in those with BRCA1 mutations and 11–17% in BRCA mutations [28, 29]. This also seems to persist in Mexican patients, with a risk of 40% for ovarian cancer in those BRCA mutations [30]. Not only BRCA mutational status is considered a risk for Ovarian cancer, but it also implicates a prognosis factor, as well as a therapeutic opportunity due to the use of poly (ADP-ribose) (PARP) inhibitors [31]. When analyzing it's prognosis value, those with BRCA1 mutational status have a worse recurrence free survival when compared with those with BRCA2 in Mexican patients with ovarian cancer [30]. This is also true when analyzing the same founder mutation, previously mentioned in the breast cancer section. Those with BRCA1 ex9–12del, which was present in (28.2%) of 179 patients analyzed compared to other BRCA1 mutations had a better recurrence free survival [30]. Knowing that BRCA mutational status has a prognosis value, this clearly reflects the necessity to have more access to BRCA tests in our population. Not only, does mutational prognosis value, but also a therapeutic opportunity. PARP inhibitors, such as Olaparib have different clinical indications, such as maintenance therapy after 1st line therapy, as well after maintenance therapy after 2 or more lines of chemotherapy [32]. In Mexico, those patients treated with Olaparib had a median progression-free survival of 12 months after 2 lines or more of chemotherapy vs. 8.3 months after 4 or more lines of chemotherapy [33]. These results are similar to what was reported in the SOLO-2 trial reporting a median progression-free survival with olaparib (19·1 months [95% CI 16·3–25·7]) than with placebo (5·5 months [5·2–5·8]; hazard ratio [HR] 0·30 [95% CI 0·22–0·41], $p < 0·0001$); there was also benefit in in overall survival of 51·7 months (95% CI 41·5–59·1) with olaparib and 38·8 months (31·4–48·6) with placebo (hazard ratio 0·74 [95% CI 0·54–1·00]; $p = 0·054$, [34, 35]. Considering the previous outcomes, it's clear why all patients which ovarian cancer, should be tested for BRCA mutational status. If a founder mutation determination is available, it should be performed. In an observational study 107 out of 377 patients were with BRCA mutation, of which 77 patients (72.9%) had BRCA1 mutation where 27.3%of these patients had the founder mutation BRCA1-Del ex9–12. When analyzing progression-free survival, patients treated with Olaparib with BRCA1-Del ex9–12 had a longer progressive free survival when compared to the rest of Mexican patients with BRCA 1 or BRCA 2 mutation treated with Olaparib [36].

4. BRCA 1/2 mutations and prostate cancer in Mexico

Although Prostate cancer is the most common cancer in Men in Mexico, [4], where those with BRCA mutational status have a higher risk of developing prostate cancer, only 1.2% to 3.2% are associated to BRCA2 mutations, even less cases to BRCA1 [37]. Although the prevalence of BRCA2 mutational status es low, it's presence is considered of poor prognosis. When compared with the general population with prostate cancer, those with BRCA2 mutation had a 12-year cancer-specific survival of 61.8% compared to 94.3% to those without BRCA2 mutation [38]. Due to its low prevalence, as well as low access to BRCA diagnosis tests, information on its impact in Mexico is scarce. In an observational study performed in a tertiary hospital in Mexico City, out of 22 patients with Castration naïve and Castration resistant prostate cancer, only 3 patients had BRCA mutational status. Contrary to global incidence, in this study BRCA1 mutational status more common than BRCA2, where all 3 patients had castration resistant prostate cancer [38]. Due to the recent approval of Olaparib in the metastatic setting in Mexico, there is not any prospective data showing its use and impact in Mexico. Even though we lack information from our population, we believe that BRCA mutational status should be determined primarily based on family history of other BRCA-related cancers.

5. Concluding remarks

As it most Latin American countries, in Mexico access to diagnosis tests is primarily an obstacle that has been resolving in the last year having more access to BRCA determination with the help of distant programs sponsored by private companies which the intention to detect which patients could benefit from PARP inhibitors. This access could help us determinate the prognosis in our population to those with BRCA mutations, as well as its impact when treated with PARP inhibitors, most of them are approved in our country. This specific population requires a directed investigation as was the case with breast and ovarian cancer where those with founder mutations had a different prognosis and response to treatment. Access not only to BRCA mutation diagnosis test, but also to founder mutations determinations is an objective that should be available in the next years to come.

Conflict of interest

The authors declare no conflict of interest.

Author details

Carlos Arturo Gonzalez Nuñez*, Paula Anel Cabrera Galeana, Sandy Ruiz Cruz and Alexandra Garcilazo Reyes
National Cancer Institute, Mexico City, Mexico

*Address all correspondence to: drgonzalez.oncologia@gmail.com

References

[1] Kim SI, Lee M, Kim HS, Chung HH, Kim JW, Park NH, et al. Effect of BRCA mutational status on survival outcome in advanced-stage high-grade serous ovarian cancer. Journal of Ovarian Research. 2019;**12**(1)

[2] Maksimenko J, Irmejs A, Nakazawa-Miklasevica M, Melbarde-Gorkusa I, Trofimovics G, Gardovskis J, et al. Prognostic role of BRCA1 mutation in patients with triple-negative breast cancer. Oncology Letters. 2014;**7**(1):278-284

[3] Huszno J, Kołosza Z, Grzybowska EWA. BRCA1 mutation in breast cancer patients: Analysis of prognostic factors and survival. Oncology Letters. 2019;**17**(2):1986-1995

[4] Sung H, Ferlay J, Siegel RL, Laversanne M, Soerjomataram I, Jemal A, et al. Global cancer statistics 2020: GLOBOCAN estimates of incidence and mortality worldwide for 36 cancers in 185 countries. CA: a Cancer Journal for Clinicians. 2021;**71**(3):209-249

[5] Mexicana G de. Tercera revisión del Consenso Nacional sobre Diagnóstico y Tratamiento del Cáncer Mamario. Available from: www.smeo.org.mx

[6] Aura D, Erazo A, Solís V. Publicación Oficial de la Sociedad Mexicana de Oncología [Internet]. Available from: www.smeo.org.mx

[7] Cárdenas-Sánchez J, Bargalló-Rocha E, Valle AE, Maafs-Molina E, Chacón AP, Clave P. Consenso Mexicano sobre Diagnóstico y Tratamiento del Cáncer Mamario [Internet]. Vol. 12. 2013. Available from: www.elsevier.es*Autorparacorrespondencia:Correoelectrónico:jesuscardenass@gmail.com.Páginadelconsenso:http://consensocancermamario.com

[8] Cáncer de mama en mujeres jóvenes en México- necesidades y retos clínicos

[9] Romero-Cordoba SL, Salido-Guadarrama I, Rebollar-Vega R, Bautista-Piña V, Dominguez-Reyes C, Tenorio-Torres A, et al. Comprehensive omic characterization of breast cancer in Mexican-Hispanic women. Nature Communications. 2021;**12**(1)

[10] Buys SS, Dickson P, Domchek SM, Elkhanany A, Friedman S, Goggins M, et al. NCCN Guidelines Version 2.2022 Genetic/Familial High-Risk Assessment: Breast, Ovarian, and Pancreatic Vanderbilt-Ingram Cancer Center [Internet]. 2022. Available from: https://www.nccn.org/home/member

[11] Paluch-Shimon S, Cardoso F, Sessa C, Balmana J, Cardoso MJ, Gilbert F, et al. Prevention and screening in BRCA mutation carriers and other breast/ovarian hereditary cancer syndromes: ESMO clinical practice guidelines for cancer prevention and screening. Annals of Oncology. 2016;**27**:v103-v110

[12] Med A, Vázquez JD, et al. Prevalencia de mutación germinal en CM www.medigraphic.org.mx INTRODUCCIÓN [Internet]. Vol. 66. 2021. Available from: www.medigraphic.org.mx

[13] Herzog JS, Chavarri-Guerra Y, Castillo D, Abugattas J, Villarreal-Garza C, Sand S, et al. Genetic epidemiology of BRCA1- and BRCA2-associated cancer across Latin America. NPJ Breast Cancer. 2021;**7**(1)

[14] Armstrong N, Ryder S, Forbes C, Ross J, Quek RGW. A systematic review

of the international prevalence of BRCA mutation in breast cancer. In: Clinical Epidemiology. Vol. 11. Dove Medical Press Ltd; 2019. pp. 543-561

[15] Larsen MJ, Kruse TA, Tan Q, Lænkholm AV, Bak M, Lykkesfeldt AE, et al. Classifications within molecular subtypes enables identification of BRCA1/BRCA2 mutation carriers by RNA tumor profiling. PLoS One. 2013;**8**(5)

[16] Weitzel JN, Clague J, Martir-Negron A, Ogaz R, Herzog J, Ricker C, et al. Prevalence and type of BRCA mutations in Hispanics undergoing genetic cancer risk assessment in the southwestern United States: A report from the clinical cancer genetics community research network. Journal of Clinical Oncology. 2013;**31**(2):210-216

[17] Villarreal-Garza C, Alvarez-Gómez RM, Pérez-Plasencia C, Herrera LA, Herzog J, Castillo D, et al. Significant clinical impact of recurrent BRCA1 and BRCA2 mutations in Mexico. Cancer. 2015;**121**(3):372-378

[18] Rashmi Kumar N, Berardi R, Abraham J, Aft R, Agnese D, Allison KH, et al. NCCN Guidelines Version 4.2022 Breast Cancer [Internet]. 2022. Available from: https://www.nccn

[19] Villarreal-Garza C, Weitzel JN, Llacuachaqui M, Sifuentes E, Magallanes-Hoyos MC, Gallardo L, et al. The prevalence of BRCA1 and BRCA2 mutations among young Mexican women with triple-negative breast cancer. Breast Cancer Research and Treatment. 2015;**150**(2):389-394

[20] Gogola E, Rottenberg S, Jonkers J. Resistance to PARP inhibitors: Lessons from preclinical models of BRCA-associated cancer. Annual Review of Cancer Biology. 2019;**3**:235-254. [Internet]. DOI: 10.1146/annurev-cancerbio-030617

[21] Tutt ANJ, Garber JE, Kaufman B, Viale G, Fumagalli D, Rastogi P, et al. Adjuvant Olaparib for patients with BRCA1- or BRCA2-mutated breast cancer. New England Journal of Medicine. 2021;**384**(25):2394-2405

[22] Tung NM, Robson ME, Ventz S, Santa-Maria CA, Nanda R, Marcom PK, et al. TBCRC 048: Phase II study of Olaparib for metastatic breast cancer and mutations in homologous recombination-related genes. Journal of Clinical Oncology. 2020;**38**:4274-4282 [Internet]

[23] Gennari A, André F, Barrios CH, Cortés J, de Azambuja E, DeMichele A, et al. ESMO clinical practice guideline for the diagnosis, staging and treatment of patients with metastatic breast cancer ☆. Annals of Oncology. 2021;**32**(12):1475-1495

[24] Litton JK, Hurvitz SA, Mina LA, Rugo HS, Lee KH, Gonçalves A, et al. Talazoparib versus chemotherapy in patients with germline BRCA1/2-mutated HER2-negative advanced breast cancer: Final overall survival results from the EMBRACA trial. Annals of Oncology. 2020;**31**(11):1526-1535

[25] Robson ME, Tung N, Conte P, Im SA, Senkus E, Xu B, et al. OlympiAD final overall survival and tolerability results: Olaparib versus chemotherapy treatment of physician's choice in patients with a germline BRCA mutation and HER2-negative metastatic breast cancer. Annals of Oncology. 2019;**30**(4):558-566

[26] Collins JM, Nordstrom BL, McLaurin KK, Dalvi TB, McCutcheon SC, Bennett JC, et al. A real-world evidence

study of CDK4/6 inhibitor treatment patterns and outcomes in metastatic breast cancer by germline BRCA mutation status. Oncology and Therapy. 2021;**9**(2):575-589

[27] García-Parra J, Dalmases A, Morancho B, Arpí O, Menendez S, Sabbaghi M, et al. Poly (ADP-ribose) polymerase inhibition enhances trastuzumab antitumour activity in HER2 overexpressing breast cancer. European Journal of Cancer. 2014;**50**(15):2725-2734

[28] Antoniou A, Pharoah PDP, Narod S, Risch HA, Eyfjord JE, Hopper JL, et al. Average risks of breast and ovarian cancer associated with BRCA1 or BRCA2 mutations detected in case series unselected for family history: A combined analysis of 22 studies. American Journal of Human Genetics. 2003;**72**:1117-1130

[29] Kuchenbaecker KB, Hopper JL, Barnes DR, Phillips KA, Mooij TM, Roos-Blom MJ, et al. Risks of breast, ovarian, and contralateral breast cancer for BRCA1 and BRCA2 mutation carriers. JAMA - Journal of the American Medical Association. 2017;**317**(23):2402-2416

[30] Gallardo-Rincón D, Álvarez-Gómez RM, Montes-Servín E, Toledo-Leyva A, Montes-Servín E, Michel-Tello D, et al. Clinical evaluation of BRCA1/2 mutation in Mexican ovarian cancer patients. Translational Oncology. 2020;**13**(2):212-220

[31] Grafodatskaya D, O'Rielly DD, Bedard K, Butcher DT, Howlett CJ, Lytwyn A, et al. Practice guidelines for BRCA1/2 tumour testing in ovarian cancer. Journal of Medical Genetics. BMJ Publishing Group. 2022

[32] Armstrong D, Alvarez R, Floor J, et al. NCCN Clinical Practice Guidelines in Oncology (NCCN Guidelines ®) NCCN.org NCCN Guidelines for Patients ® available at www.nccn.org/patients [Internet]. 2022. Available from: www.nccn.org/patients

[33] Gallardo-Rincón D, Alamilla-García G, Montes-Servín E, Morales-Vázquez F, Cano-Blanco C, Coronel-Martínez J, et al. Experiencia con el uso de olaparib en pacientes con cáncer de ovario. Gaceta Médica de México. 2019;**155**(6):585-589

[34] Pujade-Lauraine E, Ledermann JA, Selle F, Gebski V, Penson RT, Oza AM, et al. Olaparib tablets as maintenance therapy in patients with platinum-sensitive, relapsed ovarian cancer and a BRCA1/2 mutation (SOLO2/ENGOT-Ov21): A double-blind, randomised, placebo-controlled, phase 3 trial. The Lancet Oncology. 2017;**18**(9):1274-1284

[35] Poveda A, Floquet A, Ledermann JA, Asher R, Penson RT, Oza AM, et al. Olaparib tablets as maintenance therapy in patients with platinum-sensitive relapsed ovarian cancer and a BRCA1/2 mutation (SOLO2/ENGOT-Ov21): A final analysis of a double-blind, randomised, placebo-controlled, phase 3 trial. The Lancet Oncology. 2021;**22**(5):620-631

[36] Gallardo-Rincón D, Montes-Servín E, Alamilla-García G, Montes-Servín E, Bahena-González A, Cetina-Pérez L, et al. Clinical benefits of Olaparib in Mexican ovarian cancer patients with founder mutation BRCA1-Del ex9-12. Frontiers in Genetics. 2022;**13**

[37] Prevention C, Hereditary G. Epidemiology accepted on a. The Role of BRCA Testing in Hereditary Pancreatic

and Prostate Cancer Families 2019. Available from:

[38] Akbari MR, Wallis CJ, Toi A, Trachtenberg J, Sun P, Narod SA, et al. The impact of a BRCA2 mutation on mortality from screen-detected prostate cancer. British Journal of Cancer. 2014;**111**(6):1238-1240

Chapter 8

Quality of Life is Essential: Implications for Diagnosis and Treatment for BRCA1/2 Germline Mutations

Yuliana Sanchez Contreras, Brigney Isvettia Aceves Poveda, David Neri Acosta Gutierrez and Rosa Maria Alvarez Gomez

Abstract

BRCA1 and *BRCA2* germline pathogenic variants are a matter of concern because of their relevance in cancer risk assessment, personalized treatment options, and cancer prevention. Therefore, the study of quality of life (QoL), although complex, has been a challenge for clinical care and research implications for patients and families with hereditary breast and ovarian cancer (HBOC). This chapter aims to show the evolution of the evaluation of the QoL study according to the current needs of patients with *BRCA1/BRCA2* mutations.

Keywords: *BRCA1*, *BRCA2*, hereditary cancer, pathogenic variants, quality of life, risk-reducing surgeries, hereditary breast and ovarian cancer

1. Introduction

Since the discovery of germline pathogenic genes such as *BRCA1/BRCA2*, which confer high susceptibility to the development of cancer, medical care and research have been transformed in accordance with the needs of a group of people with an exceptional propensity for cancer. This has made it possible to speak in terms of risk management, such as clinical surveillance, risk-reducing surgeries, and targeted therapies, all aimed at a single goal, improving quality of life (QoL).

However, the term QoL, particularly in the medical field, has had several difficulties in its use, which make it even more difficult to evaluate. Although there is no homogeneous definition of QoL, particularly in chronic diseases such as cancer, survival plays an important role. Therefore, the evaluation of the QoL in non-modifiable conditions such as hereditary cancer implies an integral and multidisciplinary overview, in the spirit of not only influencing the gain of years lived in the course of a disease, or in the knowledge of the possibility of suffering from it, but also in the perception of well-being, which is a constant companion in the different moments of the processes of diagnosis, monitoring, treatment, and prevention.

2. Quality of life

The definition of QoL has had several fluctuations throughout history, all of them considered important from the point of view and context in which they have been used. This phenomenon of diversification in the definition could be explained due to socioeconomic, political, cultural, or philosophical circumstances. Consequently, it is likely that QoL is perceived differently [1]. However, we can identify two historical and crucial starting points, in which its study becomes relevant, and with it its incorporation into the medical field [2, 3]. The first dates from the mid-nineteenth century, with the dramatic increase in life expectancy in developed countries, and with chronic diseases began to play a leading role in public health [4]. This change, from acute infectious diseases to chronic diseases, also implies a change in perspective oriented to long-term treatment, which can undoubtedly increase life expectancy, but also its efficacy and cost-effectiveness [4, 5]. The second historical event begins with the incorporation of the term "Health", proposed by the World Health Organization (WHO) in 1948, which is "the complete state of physical, mental and social well-being and not merely the absence of disease" [6]. Later, in 1957, a WHO collaborating group proposed health as "a condition or quality" of a human organism, which expresses its adequate functioning under certain genetic or environmental conditions [6, 7].

With this preamble, the long road that researchers have traveled in search of a more homogeneous definition of the concept of QoL is framed. In 1966, within the framework of the World Health Forum held in Geneva, the WHO defined QoL as "the individual's perception of his or her position in life, within the cultural context and value system, in which he or she lives, and with respect to his or her goals, expectations, standards and interests" [8]. Under this precept, authors such as Andrews and Withey, focused their efforts on the study of QoL understood as "an effective response to one's own role situations or values" [9], giving way to a subjective area that should be considered in the study of QoL. Therefore, other aspects that determine certain conditions of the individual, such as economic, social, environmental, lifestyle, and even genetic aspects, should be considered in the study of QoL.

Given the complexity of the study of QoL derived from the objectives pursued in each investigation, the need arises to consider the term QoL as a construct, which should not only encompass aspects related to health, but also other aspects. At this point, several authors, including Cella et al., begin to outline two fundamental elements to be considered: a subjective component or "self-assessment", always measured from the subject's perspective; and the existence of external determinants that will potentially model this (objective component). Later, these determinants will give way to a multidimensional perspective in the study of QoL, as well as the areas or domains that should be included for a more complete assessment [10].

Among the multiple definitions of QoL that have been proposed over time, two major difficulties have become evident: a) lack of consensus or homogeneity in the definition and b) how to measure QoL [3, 11, 12].

Certainly, this problem has contributed to the use of terms such as "well-being", "Health-Related Quality of Life" (HRQoL) and even identified as "synonyms" of QoL. Thus, several authors frame the dynamic course of the study of QoL not only according to the context in which it is assessed but also from the time and area of study, considering QoL as the difference between the subject's functional level and the ideal standard [1, 10–12].

Nowadays cancer is conceptualized as a chronic disease, thanks to improvements in medical care and treatments. The study of QoL has run in parallel, seeking to better understand patients' perceptions in the spheres of physical, mental, family, and cultural health [13].

For a long time, QoL was considered as a term homologous to survival, assessing the outcome of the disease in purely numerical terms. However, it did not show the disease patient's process. Therefore, it is essential to evaluate QoL from the patient's perception, and not exclusively from the medical perspective, without losing the objective of a measurement with the aim of reducing symptoms and prolonging life [13].

In order to better understand why survival was long considered QoL, we must focus on the process of medical care received by an oncology patient, which differs from other chronic diseases. The first point is the news of the diagnosis, which involves intense emotions of shock, fear, anger, and anxiety. All of them are evoked by one word: "cancer" [14]. The second factor is "how advanced" the disease is, the clinical stage at diagnosis. This step is a crucial event since medical and surgical management will depend on its evaluation. The choice between "conservative" treatment, or the therapeutic "arsenal" of surgery-chemotherapy-radiotherapy, is a challenge for the patient, with an important emotional burden that can trigger psychiatric disorders [15].

There is ample evidence of the high frequency of anxiety and depression in cancer patients, with a frequency ranging between 10 and 20%, which is a 2 to 3 times higher risk than in the general population [16, 17]. Psychiatric symptoms triggered by the disease can negatively affect QoL [18, 19]. Therefore, Lara and collaborators [13], consider as crucial the evaluation of QoL, as part of the care before and after each intervention in cancer. Thus, QoL will fulfill its objective of being "the most sensitive and powerful measure of the results of treatments or interventions" [20] and will make it possible to identify the adaptations that each patient needs to make in the physical, psychological, family, work, social, economic and personal spheres. In this sense, the most widely used instrument in QoL, as it covers most of these aspects [21].

In this sense, it is important to consider not only the disease and its impact on the individual's health per se, but also the implications at the personal, family, and social levels, such as those faced by a vulnerable group, as the subgroup of patients who are carriers of germline variants. According to the definition of vulnerability provided by the United Nations Disaster Risk Reduction (UNDRR) in 2009, it refers to the characteristics and circumstances of a community or system that make it susceptible to the harmful effects of a hazard [22]. According to Tierney et al., the hazard is the agent or medium through which damage and loss can occur. Therefore, a definition of hazard contemplates natural, anthropogenic, and even a combination of both [22]. In this sense, the hereditary cancer group has a genetic condition, which increases their risk of suffering or developing cancer, making this non-modifiable factor an additional burden in various aspects, to manage this vulnerability, as mentioned by Kuran et al., depends in turn on access to and control of different resources. Assuming this, we cannot view vulnerability as a dichotomous aspect, since this group faces decision-making, and detailed planning to manage and adapt to long-term genetic risk [3, 23].

Considering this background, we can say that QoL as a construct should be measured from different perspectives, always contemplating the patient's ideals, as well as medical, personal, psychological, social, and even economic situations that may be involved in the modeling of the disease and that will influence QoL (**Figure 1**: Areas of quality of life assessment in patients with *BRCA1/BRCA2* germline pathogenic variants.

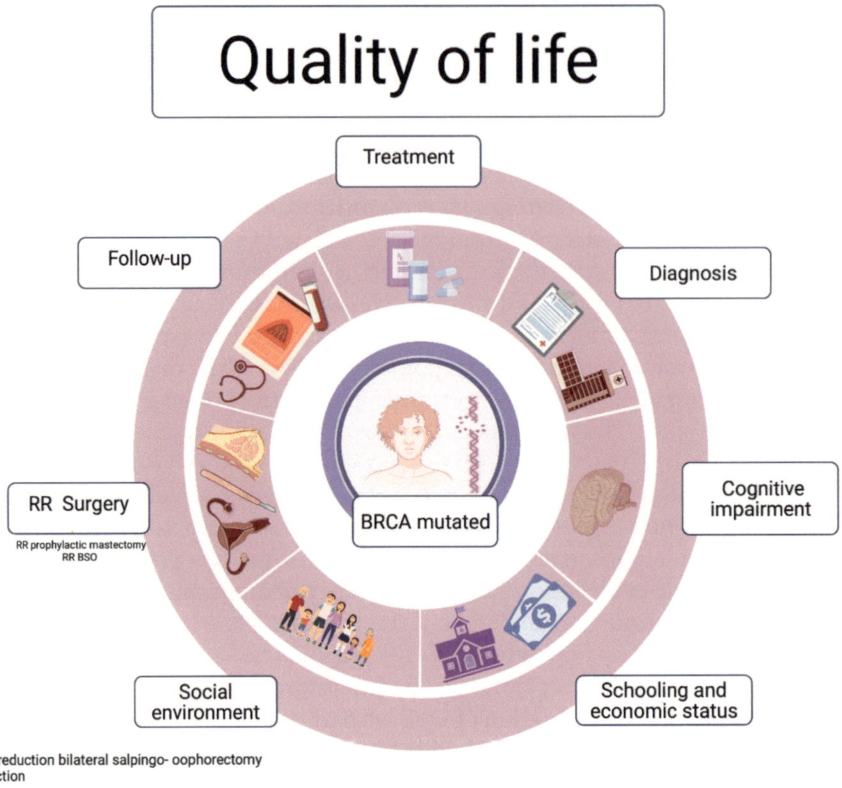

Figure 1.
Quality of life in patients that have a cancer diagnosis with BRCA genes pathogenic variants, has a meaningful repercussion in different aspects that construct life. This type of diagnosis represents a more periodic follow-up plan, including the option of risk reduction surgeries that can be a difficult decision and complex process. Adding to the previous, the possibility of inheritance to a family can increase anxiety, and have a negative impact on the patient's cognitive understanding and coping with information. All these aspects must be evaluated for a multidisciplinary assessment.

3. Quality of life in patients carrying mutations in *BRCA1 /BRCA2*

For a better understanding of the circumstances surrounding *BRCA1/BRCA2* germline pathogenic variants carriers, we need to know about the genetic context of what the term "pathogenic variant" or "mutation" implies, and why it has become a watershed for oncology, genetics, and research. In this sense, since the discovery of the cancer susceptibility related to *BRCA1* [24] and *BRCA2* [25] genes, a new perspective on conceived cancer has emerged. The BRCA genes are tumor suppressors with remarkable participation in the maintenance of genomic stability by promoting the repair of DNA double-strand breaks, by the Homologous Recombination (HR) pathway [26, 27]. The phenotype attributable, hereditary breast and ovarian cancer syndrome (HBOC), is the most studied hereditary cancer [28–30]. HBOC patients have a 60 to 80% risk of developing breast cancer, and a 16 to 45% risk of developing ovarian cancer [31–33]. Therefore, it is so important to diagnose it on time, as well as to provide care and prevention. This increased risk in this population led to the creation of groups of experts and international criteria like one of the National Comprehensive Cancer Network (NCCN), in its most recent version 2.2021 [34], which allows early identification and referral.

Research groups have directed their efforts not only to the identification of this population, but also in comprehensive care, that is, to all those areas involved in medical-psychological care (medical oncologists, surgical oncologists, geneticists, gynecologic oncologists, and oncological psychology). This comprehensive model has made evident opportunity areas with important contributions to the understanding of the health-disease process of this population, and the effect that hereditary cancer has on their QoL [33, 35, 36].

We recognize the variety of treatment schemes (surgery, chemotherapy, radiotherapy, hormone therapy, etc.) that oncology patients usually go through in their care process [37–41]. For this reason, Goerling et al. [21] state the importance of QoL study in the oncology patient, in which the different stages that the patient experiences throughout the process must be contemplated [21]. Ganz et al. describe the existence of non-medical factors that should be evaluated, such as QoL, since they have an impact on survival, and therefore should be considered as predictors of survival [42]. However, in the patient with hereditary cancer, there is an added emotional and stressful burden of knowing that she/he is a carrier of a germline variant, which increases the risk of cancer, with the possibility of being able to pass it on to offspring, a very important factor that is mostly evidenced in young women [43].

Current studies in the hereditary cancer population who undergo a genetic test, have shown increased symptoms of anxiety, depression, and stress related to the risk of suffering or developing cancer. These symptoms are even more prevalent in women who have had a cancer family history, or who have lived the experience of being the primary caregiver of a family member with cancer [43–45].

The crucial role of genetic counseling is becoming increasingly clear since it is considered a communication process for the "translation of genetic information", into words that can be understood and managed with respect to genetic risk. For this reason, the information provided not only affects the individual in question but also influences the rest of the family [46, 47].

Given this situation, it is central to emphasize the personalization of genetic counseling. According to Wenzel et al. [48], they show that people who have had personal experience of cancer have a greater adaptation to communication related to the increased risk of being a carrier, compared to the general population. However, the news given in genetic counseling are perceived with an additional psychological, emotional, social, and health load. Likewise, those women who have witnessed the death of one or more relatives because of cancer have reported greater difficulty in adjusting to the loss [48]. Thus, the QoL is significantly lower for those who have suffered the loss of a close relative, such as parents, compared to those who have not had this loss.

In addition, it is also significant to consider the "asymptomatic" state of individuals who undergo genetic testing, since it has been shown that the risk is not perceived in the same way, in comparison with those who have suffered cancer. Asymptomatic carriers perceive it as a "duality", whether they have the risk or not, and therefore decisions regarding risk management (risk-reducing surgeries or clinical surveillance), are postponed or anticipated, generating a considerable increase in anxiety, stress and anguish, and even, avoidance [48, 49].

Considering this panorama, it is essential to provide genetic counseling, so that the patient can have complete, reliable, available, and manageable information that allows them to manage the risk for their own benefit, even extending it to their family. Likewise, the emotional, psychological, and social weight of being a mutation carrier must be considered, since the environment in which the patient lives is crucial for the economic, social adaptations, and decisions [46, 48, 50].

4. Effects on quality of life in the risk care of patients carrying mutations in *BRCA1 /BRCA2*

As we have been able to appreciate, the implications of a "tiny" change in the sequence of our genetic material can cause major events in the daily life of a person. The identification of this population has made it possible to contribute to the improvement of surveillance strategies, treatments, and preventive measures, intending to reduce cancer risk and preserving life [34, 51].

The strategies will be divided into two large groups: clinical surveillance (CS) and risk-reducing surgeries (RRS). Within the first group, all those laboratory or cabinet studies that will allow surveillance of target organs are prone to the development of cancer. These studies include mammography, magnetic resonance imaging, a transvaginal ultrasound, and tumor markers, such as Ca-125 [34, 52].

For the second group, two surgical events are considered that have the purpose of removing the target organ, breasts, and/or ovaries, called risk-reducing mastectomy (RRM), in its contralateral or bilateral presentation; and risk-reducing bilateral salpingo-oophorectomy (RRBSO) [33, 53–55]. Both surgeries are cost-effective for long-term risk management [56–58].

4.1 Risk-reducing surgeries

To date, there is robust evidence of the risk reduction benefits of risk-reducing surgery, both RRM and RRBSO [59–61].

4.1.1 Risk-reducing mastectomy (RRM): contralateral or bilateral

When speaking of RRM, since 1998, there is a record of an increase in the rates of performing this surgery, a factor that possibly led to this increase was the so-called "Jolie effect" [62], in which an American actress, carrier of a *BRCA* pathogenic variant, opted for RRM. This phenomenon was widely discussed in various studies, in which the point of discussion was the pertinence of surgery, as well as the indications and the short- and long-term effects [63, 64].

Part of this evidence has made it possible to visualize that the performance of this surgery implies a reduction of at least up to 90% of the risk of developing breast cancer [33, 65]. Similarly, it has been documented the existence of medical and other factors, which may be associated with and influence the decision-making regarding its performance. These factors have been specifically described as: the accessibility to immediate breast reconstruction for aesthetic purposes; economic costs; recovery time, and the age of the patient at the time of the intervention. The average age estimated in the RRM performance was 36. 5–41 years [66], a condition that corroborates Filippo et al., stating that decision-making is more complex in premenopausal patients, among others. Likewise, this type of risk intervention had physical repercussions: infections, bleeding, lymphedema, chronic pain, and/or discomfort of the sensitive type in the surgical area, contracture, or rejection of the implant, among others [65].

As we have seen, researchers became concerned not only with the physical effects derived from the surgical procedure but also began to evaluate them from the perspective of the psychological effect [33, 67]. Among these aspects, the most evaluated were stress, depression and anxiety, all of them in relation to cancer risk, and/or the cosmetic results of risk-reducing surgery [68]. The results obtained reveal significantly high levels of stress and anxiety perceived before surgery. However, these decreased after surgery. It is also revealed that, despite some dissatisfaction with the aesthetic results, most of the women who choose an RRM, considered themselves satisfied with the decision [33, 65, 68, 69]. Another important factor to evaluate in these studies was the effect on sexuality, obtaining results without statistically significant differences when compared with the general population [68].

It is worth mentioning that, in most of these studies, the objective has been HRQoL and not general QoL. Therefore, it is important to point out that despite the increase of RRM after the "Jolie effect", this surgery continues to be less accepted in comparison with RRBSO, since the latter is associated with a lower rate of complications, as well as a shorter recovery time [33, 65].

4.1.2 Risk-Reducing Bilateral Salpingo-Oophorectomy (RRBSO)

This surgical measure involves a reduction in the risk of ovarian cancer described in up to 95% women who are carriers of pathogenic variants in *BRCA1/BRCA2* [33, 68, 70, 71].

As with RRM, this type of intervention had to undergo several studies to demonstrate the correlation between its implementation and risk reduction [70]. This path also involved a study focused only on physical aspects or adverse events [33, 71, 72]. These studies also describe these effects and above all how they affect mostly young women [<40 years], such as early menopause, osteoporosis derived from estrogen suppression, decreased libido, and another factor of even greater concern, fertility [73, 74].

RRBSO is one of the most widely accepted risk-reducing surgeries for this at-risk population [33, 70–72]. According to the NCCN [34], this surgery is recommended in women whose parity has been satisfied, and it is also indicated in an estimated age range between 35 and 40 years [70, 71].

Among the effects described that exerted effect in areas related to HRQoL, were similar in various populations, such as shorter recovery time (if this was performed with surgical techniques that involved less invasive as laparoscopy), decreased libido, vaginal dryness, and vasomotor signs (night sweats and "hot flashes"), that would be treated with hormone replacement therapy [33, 70, 74]. Also, it has been reported, a significant increase in stress and anxiety before surgery, that decrease after the surgical event [33, 74–77].

As we have seen, both surgical events have robust evidence of their contribution to the reduction of cancer risk; however, a factor to highlight in both is the criticism of the lack of medical information describing the effects related to their performance, the times at which they should be performed, recovery times, and especially for RRM, esthetic results [33, 65]. Despite this, the acceptance rates of these forms of risk management are high in the *BRCA1/BRCA2* carrier populations [65, 70, 73]. In this sense, it is important to highlight that there is indiscriminate use of the terms QoL and HRQoL [68], as mentioned by Haraldstad et al. [1], in their systematic review on QoL research in medicine, a point of view that highlights the long road that still lies ahead in the study of QoL, and all those factors associated [1].

Razdan et al. show that although high levels of "general well-being", "body image" and HRQoL are maintained, methodological rigor must also be considered, which will allow the inclusion of other instruments that will allow the desired objectives to be achieved in the evaluation of general QoL [68].

4.2 Clinical surveillance (CV)

This type of risk management strategy involves the performance laboratories and radiological images for timely detection of cancer [33, 34, 43, 51–54, 56, 58]. Likewise, due to the "difficulty" of following patients over time, this type of study has not yielded robust evidence of a decrease in the specific risk associated, as in the case of risk-reducing surgeries. What we know today is that this type of screening involves detection in the very early stages of breast cancer specifically. However, there is a lack of studies with a close surveillance methodology for ovarian cancer [52, 78].

Particularly in this group of QoL, a significant increase in stress levels experienced by women has been documented, before medical consultation, in relation to the results of follow-up studies. [33, 34, 52]. Another non-medical aspect is the cost of surveillance studies, since these are performed regularly, and this implies an increase in expenses compared to patients who only have surveillance without adding the genetic factor, or those who opted for risk-reducing surgery. Similar data in other populations, where the RRM is less frequent, it is associated with a higher rate of surgical complications; immediate, mediate, and late, reflected as cosmetic results not well accepted by the patients [79, 80]. Other authors have evidenced the inconformity of the patients for receiving "little" information about the possible medical and cosmetic results of RRM, since by receiving more information, they would have more opportunity to weigh the complications and adversities they would face with a procedure of this nature [33, 69].

5. Quality of life: comparison between the two risk management strategies

Perhaps the question at this point is: Which care strategy is best for people with *BRCA* gene mutations, in terms of QoL? While it is true that both offer risk management, both have advantages and disadvantages. It is imperative to always consider the patient's decision. As we have seen in the first lines of this chapter, talking about QoL is not a dichotomous answer but a more complex one that allows us to contemplate factors that we do not essentially see at first glance, but that will be a fundamental part of the modeling and course of the disease, in this case, cancer surveillance and its risk management.

It is somewhat tempting to assume that one risk intervention is better than the other; however, there is evidence to support that according to the population and its context, both can be feasible options, since when both strategies were compared in different populations, the levels of QoL and HRQoL did not show a statistically significant difference [75, 76, 78]. An important fact to be highlighted in these studies comparing both strategies is the instruments used for measurement, their validation, the objectives, and, above all, the areas evaluated [1]. Likewise, it is important to consider, as mentioned by Razdan et al. the objectives and methodological strategies of each research. Therefore, talking about QoL and risk management strategies in this population is still a challenge in medical research and an area of opportunity.

6. Effects on quality of life of target therapies: PARP inhibitors for HBOC patients

Throughout the history of medicine, we have been able to corroborate the great advances that have been made in different therapies that have marked the course of our history, from antibiotic therapy and the implementation of vaccines to the present day where a small change can be the distinction and the "target" for new therapies. Such is the case of the drugs that have caused a great revolution in oncology, the poly (adenosine diphosphate [ADP]-ribose) polymerase (PARP) inhibitors (iPARP) [81, 82].

These types of therapies aim to interfere with specific molecules, block signals that favor cancer cell growth, interfere with cell cycle regulation, as well as induce cell death, preventing cancer progression [83], making them the first drugs targeting the response to DNA damage to be used in the treatment of cancer patients [81, 82] (**Figure 2**: Mechanism of action of PARP inhibitors).

Nowadays, cancer hallmarks are known such as maintaining proliferation signals, allowing cell immortality, stimulating nutrient supply to tumors, and evasion of the immune system, among others, which will allow uncontrolled and abnormal cell growth [84], therefore, anticancer drugs have been designed to target the entire panel of cancer hallmarks [81].

To date, four iPARPs, olaparib, talazoparib, rucaparib, and niraparib, have been approved by the Food and Drug Administration (FDA), and the European Medicines Agency (EMA) [81, 85] for the treatment of patients with breast, ovarian, prostate, and pancreas cancer.

These drugs have become an important axis in the treatment of patients with breast and ovarian cancer. Nevertheless, their study and effect on patients carrying mutations in genes such as *BRCA1/BRCA2* have been more relevant. Their importance lies in

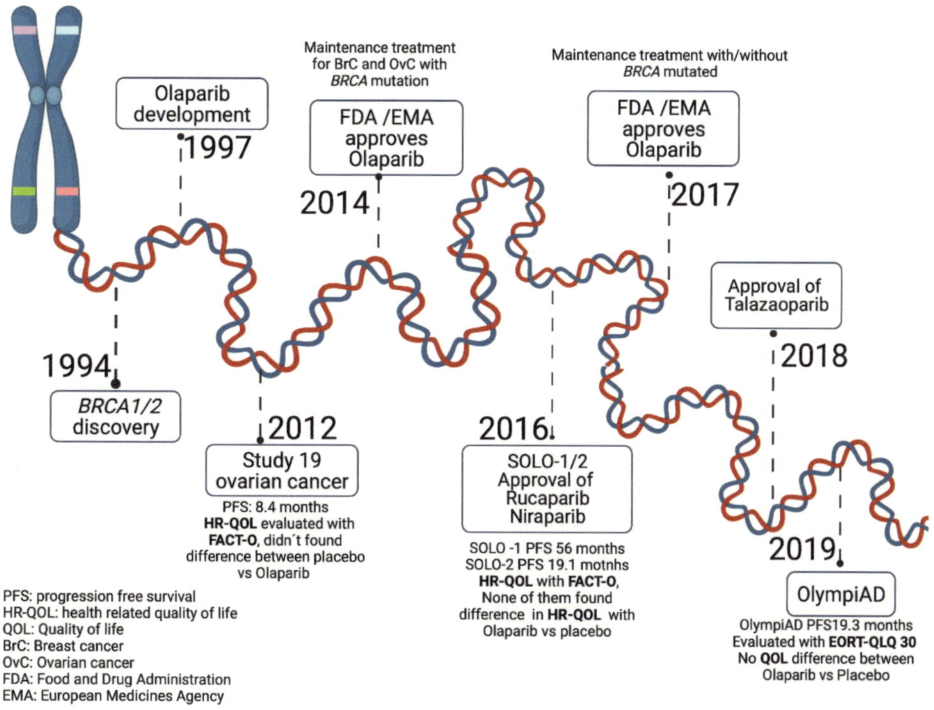

Figure 2.
(A) Normal SSBRS: PARP detects the single strand break in DNA, marking the point for the SSBRS to restore the genetic information; and (B) Olaparib treatment: Olaparib inhibits the PARP protein prolonging its repair. Eventually, the second strand of DNA will be damaged. If BRCA is mutated, the cell will be unable to repair a "double strand break", making the only way to lead to cell death.

Year	Milestone/Clinical Trial	Important events
1994	*BRCA1/2* discovery	• Association with the development of breast and ovarian cancer. (Ref)
1997	Olaparib development	
2012	Study 19	• Focus on ovarian cancer
		• PFS was significantly longer with Olaparib (8.4 months) [1].
		• HRQoL measure with FACT-O
		• No difference between placebo vs Olaparib [1].
		• Treatment with Olaparib was well tolerated and had no adverse impact on HRQoL [2].
2014	FDA/EMA approval for Olaparib	• Maintenance treatment for breast and ovarian cancer with *BRCA* mutation
2016	SOLO-1 SOLO-2	• SOLO-1 PFS was 56 months with Olaparib [3].
		• Maintenance therapy with Olaparib provided a substantial benefit to PFS [4].
		• SOLO-2 PFS was 19.1 months with Olaparib [6].
		• HRQoL with FACT-O in SOLO-2, Olaparib maintenance therapy did not have a significant detrimental effect on HRQoL compared with placebo [5].
2016	FDA approval Niraparib and Rucaparib	• Advanced ovarian cancer [8]
2017	FDA/EMA approval for Olaparib	• Maintenance treatment with/without *BRCA* mutated
2018	Approval of Talazoparib	• Germline BRCA-mutated locally advance or metastatic breast cancer
2019	OlympiAD	• PFS was 7 months versus chemotherapy treatment of physician's choice [7].
		• QoL measure with EORT-QLQ 30
		• No difference between placebo vs Olaparib

Table 1.
Important events around iPARP.

the fact that these genes, also known as "tumor suppressor", are part of a surveillance system that helps to control cell multiplication, as well as repair DNA double-strand breaks through a process known as homologous recombination (HR), thus allowing DNA integrity [81, 86]. In patients with mutations in these tumor suppressor genes, this surveillance system is affected, contributing to a key part of the action of these targeted drugs, since IPARPs disable another DNA damage repair mechanism called "PAR-ylation", achieving a break in the first DNA strand and breaking the second strand at this point in the process, However, in patients carrying pathogenic mutations in these genes, this repair process becomes almost impossible, leading the cell to what we call "synthetic lethality", i.e., it forces a highly damaged cell to imminent death to prevent its proliferation and thus perpetuate the damage [87–89].

Knowing in broad strokes the mechanism of action of these drugs, we can understand their relevance in this population. For this reason, since their discovery, several clinical trials have been carried out to determine not only their effectiveness but also the adverse effects of their administration, the doses at which they work, and, above all, the objective response rate, which refers to the reduction in tumor size after treatment, showing mostly satisfactory results in patients with *BRCA1/BRCA2* mutations [90–104].

This last factor of interest, as we have already mentioned in the first lines of this chapter, survival has been used as a synonym of HRQoL [4, 5]. Therefore, there is ample and robust evidence from clinical trials, where instruments have been used for the evaluation of HRQoL, well-being, and symptomatology, in general without obtaining statistically significant results that allow us to differentiate whether these patients carrying mutations, who benefit from a targeted therapy that increases their median progression-free survival, present optimal levels of QoL when compared with other standard therapies such as chemotherapy [105, 106].

One of the most widely used drugs today is Olaparib, which is approved by the FDA and EMA for patients with advanced ovarian cancer as maintenance therapy independent of *BRCA1/BRCA2* status [101, 102], which in clinical trials has demonstrated an increase in progression-free survival estimated at 13. 8 months to 49.9 months, compared to placebo (standard therapy) which was 5.5–19.1 months, this fact is of utmost importance to clinicians as the goal of life-sustaining is pursued. However, it has also been shown that the study of QoL in these patients and especially in this type of research, continues to be a subject to development, because HRQoL is still evaluated as a synonym of QoL, [105, 106]. **Table 1** key events in the development of PARP inhibitors and quality of life.

Likewise, this lack of an operational definition, as shown by Razdan et al. has allowed the use of various instruments that only assess HRQoL, so there is still a long way to go in this type of research, with the aim of continuing to provide better and more efficient and comprehensive medical care (**Figure 3** shows transcendent events in the history of the iPARPs).

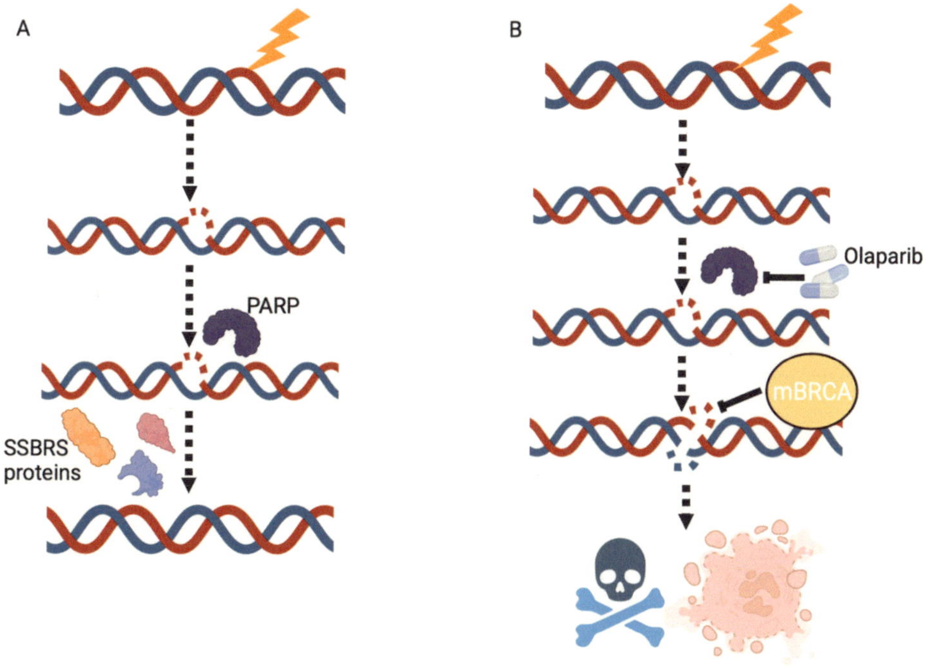

Figure 3.
This timeline represents the most important events around PARP inhibitors. From the discovery of BRCA1and BRCA2 genes and its association with the risk of developing cancer to the most relevant clinical trials that have shown an increase in the survival for this population, and how the quality of life has been evaluated in each of them.

7. Concluding remarks and perspectives

The complex concept of QoL encompasses aspects of physical, emotional, social, and cultural well-being, which may be particular to an individual. In people with increased susceptibility to cancer, for instance, carriers of germline pathogenic variants in *BRCA1* and *BRCA2* genes, the analysis of QoL presents a broad picture, involving not only the experience of cancer and its effect on one's life. It also involves family aspects, decision-making about risk reduction actions, and the perception of their repercussions, as in the case of surgeries (RRM and RRBSO).

The emergence of targeted treatments, such as PARP inhibitors, has brought to the field of the study of QoL new questions about the effects of pharmacological treatments in the context of patients with exceptional characteristics in their oncologic pathway.

As it has been pointed out by several authors in the field, it will be necessary to continue with the research of QoL in this group of patients and families, with the indispensable adaptations that will allow to dimension as broadly as possible the nature of the phenomenon.

Acknowledgements

We thank the patients and families of the Hereditary Cancer Clinic of the National Cancer Institute for their participation in the research projects, which inspire us to build better answers to their concerns and optimize their medical care.

We also thank the LXV legislature of the Chamber of Deputies for the budget allocation for program 309 "Hereditary Cancer Clinic".

Conflict of interest

The authors declare no conflict of interest.

Author details

Yuliana Sanchez Contreras[1], Brigney Isvettia Aceves Poveda[1], David Neri Acosta Gutierrez[2] and Rosa Maria Alvarez Gomez[1*]

1 Hereditary Cancer Clinic. Nacional institute of Cancer, Mexico City, Mexico

2 Regional Hospital "Lic. Adolfo Lopez Mateos", ISSSTE, Mexico City, Mexico

*Address all correspondence to: ralvarezg@incan.edu.mx

References

[1] Haraldstad K, Wahl A, Andenaes R, Andersen JR, Andersen MH, Beisland E, et al. A systematic review of quality-of-life research in medicine and health sciences. Quality of life research: An international journal of quality-of-life aspects of treatment, care and rehabilitation. Quality of Life Research. 2019;**28**(10):2641-2650. DOI: 10.1007/s11136-09-02214-9

[2] Alfonso U, Caqueo-Urízar A. Quelity of life: Theoretical review. Ter Psicologia. 2012;**30**(1):61-71. DOI:10.4067/S0718-48082012000100006

[3] Karimi M, Brazier J. Health-related quality of life, and quality of life: What is the difference? PharmacoEconomics. 2016;**34**:645-649

[4] Katz S. The science of quality of life. Journal of Chronic Diseases. 1987;**40**(6):459-463. DOI: 10.1016/0021-9681(87)9001-4

[5] Fries JF. Aging, natural death, and the compression of morbidity. The New England Journal of Medicine. 1980;**303**(3):130-135. DOI: 10.1056/NEJM198007173030304

[6] Larson JS. The World Health Organizations definition of health: Social versus spiritual health. Social Indicator Research. 1996;**38**:181-192

[7] World Health Organization. Study Group on the Measurement of Levels of Health &World Health Organization. Measurement of levels of health: Report of a study group. [meeting held in Genova from 24 to 28 October 1955] WHO Technical Report Series. 1957

[8] Post MW. Definitions of quality of life: What has happened and how to move on. Topics in Spinal Cord Injury Rehabilitation. 2014;**20**(3):167-180. DOI: 10.1310/sci2003-167

[9] Andrews F, Withey S. Developing measures of perceived life quality: Results from several national surveys. Social Indicators Research. 1974;**1**:1-26. DOI: 10.1007/BF00286419

[10] Cella DF. Quality of life: Concepts and definition. Journal of Pain and Symptom Management. 1994;**9**(3):186-192. DOI: 10.1016/0885_3924(94)90129-5

[11] Leplège A, Hunt S. The problem of quality of life in medicine. JAMA. 1997;**278**(1):47-50. DOI: 10.1001/jama.1997.03550010061041

[12] Murri R, Fantoni M, Ortona L. Defining and measuring quality of life in medicine. JAMA. 1998;**279**(6):449

[13] Lara MC, Ponce de León S, De la Fuente JR. Conceptualización y medición de la calidad de vida en pacientes con cáncer. Revista de Investigación Clínica. 1995;**47**(4):325-327

[14] Cordova MJ, Riba MB, Spiegel D. Post-traumatic stress disorder and cancer. Lancer Psychiatry. 2017;**4**(4):330-338. DOI: 10.1016/S2215-0366(17)30014-7

[15] Smith HR. Depression in cancer patients: Pathogenesis, implications and treatment (Review). Oncological Letters. 2015;**9**(4):1509-1514

[16] Wilson K, Chochinov H, Skirko M, Allard P, Chary S, Gargnon P, et al. Depression and anxiety disorders in palliative cancer care. Journal of Pain and Symptom Management. 2007;**33**(2):118-129. DOI: 10.1016/j.jpainsymman.2006.07.016

[17] Watts S, Prescott P, Mason J, McLeod N, Lewith G. Depression and anxiety in ovarian cancer: A systematic review and meta-analysis of prevalence rates. BMJ Open. 2015;**5**(11):e007618. DOI: 10.1136/bmjopen-2015-007618

[18] Barrera TL, Norton PJ. Quality of life impairment in generalized anxiety disorder, social phobia, and panic disorder. Journal of Anxiety Disorders. 2009;**23**(8):1086-1090. DOI: 10.1016/j.janxdis.2009.07.011

[19] Kolovos S, Kleiboer A, Cuijpers P. Effect psychotherapy for depression on quality of life: Meta-analysis. The British Journal of Psychiatry. 2016;**209**(6):460-468. DOI: 10.1192/bjp.bp.115.175059

[20] Wiklund I, Lindvall K, Swedberg K. Assesment of quality of life in clinical trials. Acta Medica Scandinavica. 1986;**220**(1):1-3. DOI: 10.1111/j.0954-6820.1986.tb02723.x

[21] Goerling U, Stickel A. Quality of life in oncology. Recent Results in Cancer Research. 2014;**197**:137-152. DOI: 10.1007/978-3-642-40187-9_10

[22] Kuran CH, Morsut C, Kruke B, Krüger M, Segnestam L, Orru K, et al. Vulnerability and vulnerable groups from an intersectionality perspective. International Journal of Disaster Risk Reduction. 2020;**50**:101826. DOI: 10.1016/j.ijdrr.2020.101912

[23] Baider L, Ever-Hadani P, Kaplan D-NA. Psychological distress in healthy women with familial breast cancer: Like mother, like daughter? International Journal of Psychiatry in Medicine. 1999;**29**(4):411-420. DOI: 10.2190/LD2F-ND7R-19JK-WL4G

[24] Miki Y, Swensen J, Shattuck-Eidens D, Futreal P, Harshman K, Tavtigian S, et al. A strong candidate for the breast and ovarian cancer susceptibility gene BRCA1. Science. 1994;**266**(5182):66-71

[25] Wooster R, Neuhausen SL, Mangion J, Quirk Y, Ford D, Collins N, et al. Localization of a breast cancer susceptibility gene, BRCA2, to chromosome 13q12-13. Science. 1994;**265**(5181):2088-2090. DOI: 10.1126/science.8091231

[26] Prakash R, Zhang Y, Feng W, Jasin M. Homologus recombination and human health: The roles of BRCA1, BRCA2, and associated proteins. Cold Spring Harbor Perspectives in Biology. 2015;**7**(4):a016600. DOI: 10.1101/cshperspect.a016600

[27] Gudmundsdottir K, Ashworth A. The roles of BRCA1 and BRCA2 and associated proteins in the maintenance of genomic stability. Oncogene. 2006;**25**(43):5864

[28] Wang YA, Jian JW, Hung CF, Peng HP, Yang CH, Skye HC, et al. Germline breast cancer susceptibility gene mutations and breas cancer outcomes. BMC Cancer. 2018;**18**(1):315. DOI: 10.1186/s12885-018-4229-5

[29] Slavin T, Maxwell K, Lilyquist J, Vijai J, Neuhausen S, Hart S, et al. The contribution of pathogenic variants in breast cancer susceptibility genes to familial breast cancer risk. NPJ Breast Cancer. 2017;**3**:22. DOI: 10.1038/s41523-017-0024-8

[30] Baretta Z, Mocellin S, Goldin E, Olopade O, Huo D. Effect of BRCA germline mutations on breast cancer prognosis: A systematic review and meta-analysis. Medicine (Baltimore). 2017;**95**(40):e4975. DOI: 10.1097/MD.0000000000004975

[31] Garber J, Offit K. Hereditary cancer predisposition syndromes. Journal of

Clinical Oncology. 2005;**23**(2):276-292. DOI: 10.1200/JCO.2005.10.042

[32] Castéra L, Krieger S, Rousselin A, Legros A, Baumann J, Bruet O, et al. Next-generation sequencing for the diagnosis of hereditary breast and ovarian cancer using genomic capture targeting multiple candidate genes. European Human Genetics. 2014;**22**(11):1305-1313. DOI: 10.1038/ejhg.2014.16

[33] Alonzo M, Piva E, Pecchio S, Liberale V, Modaffari P, Ponzone R, et al. Satisfaction and impact on quality of life of clinical and instrumental surveillance and prophylactic surgery in BRCA-mutation carriers. Clinical Breast Cancer. 2018;**18**(6):e1361-e1366. DOI: 10.1016/j.clbc.2018.07.015

[34] Daly MB, Pilarski R, Yurgelun MB, Berry MP, Buys SS, Dickson P, et al. Genetic/familial high-risk assessment: Breast and ovarian and pancreatic clinical practice guidelines. Journal of the National Comprenhensive Cancer Network. 2020;**18**(4):380-391. DOI: 10.6004/jnccn.2020.0017

[35] Yoshida R. Hereditary breast and ovarian cancer (HBOC): Review of its molecular characteristics, screening, treatment, and prognosis. Breast Cancer. 2021;**28**(6):1167-1180. DOI: 10.1007/s12282-020-01148-2

[36] DiCastro M, Frydman M, Friedman I, Shiri-Sverdlov R, Papa M, Boleslaw G, et al. American Journal of Medical Genetics. 2002;**111**(2):147-151. DOI: 10.1002/ajmg.10550

[37] Orr B, Edwards R. Diagnosis and treatment of ovarian cancer. Hematology/Oncology Clinics of North America. 2018;**32**(6):943-964. DOI: 10.1016/j.hoc.2018.07.010

[38] Yang C, Xia BR, Zhang Z, Zhang Y, Lou G, Jin W. Immunotherapy for Ovarian Cancer: Adjuvant, Combination, and Neoadjuvant. Frontiers in Immunology. 2020;**11**:577869. DOI: 10.3389/fimmu.2020.577869

[39] McDonald E, Clark A, Tchou J, Zhang P, Freedman G. Clinical diagnosis and management of breast cancer. Journal of Nuclear Medicine. 2016;**57**(Suppl. 1):9S-16S. DOI: 10.2967/jnumed.115.157834

[40] Tesch M, Patridge A. Treatment of breast cancer in young adults. American Society of Clinical Oncology Educational Book. 2022;**42**:1-12. DOI: 10.1200/EDBK_360970

[41] Thoppil J, Ramya P. An overview on breast cancer genetics and recent innovations: Literature survey. Breast Disease. 2021;**40**(3):143-154. DOI: 10.3233/BD-201040

[42] Ganz P, Lee J, Siau J. Quality of life assessment. An independent prognostic variable for survival in lung cancer. Cancer. 1991;**67**(12):3131-3135

[43] Meiser B, Halliday J. What is the impact of genetic counselling in women at increased risk of developing hereditary breast cancer? A meta-analytic review. Social Science & Medicine. 2002;**54**(10):1463-1470. DOI: 10.1016/s0277-9536(01)00133-2

[44] Vodermaier A, Stanton A. Familial breast cancer: Less emotional distress in adult daughters if they provide emotional support to their affected mother. Familial Cancer. 2012;**11**(4):645-652. DOI: 10.1007/s10689-012-9566-y

[45] Valdimarsdottir H, Bovbjerg D, Kash K, Holland J, Osborne M, Miller D. Psychological distress in women with a familiar risk of breast cancer. Psychology Oncology. 1995;**4**(2):133-141

[46] Carlsson A, Bjorvatn C, Engebretsen L, Berglund G, Natvig G. Psychosocial factor

associated with quality of life among individuals attending genetic counseling for hereditary cancer. Journal of Genetic Counseling. 2004;**13**(5):425-445. DOI: 10.1023/B:JOGC.0000044202.95768.b3

[47] Hansson M. Ethical management of hereditary cancer information. Acta Oncologica. 1999;**38**(3):305-308. DOI: 10.1080/028418699431366

[48] Wenzel L, Osann K, Lester J, Kurz R, Hsieh S, Nelson E, et al. Biopsychological stress factors in BRCA mutation carriers. Psychosomatics. 2012;**53**(6):582-590. DOI: 10.1016/j.psym.2012.06.007

[49] Miller S. Monitoring versus blunting styles of coping with cancer influence the information patients want and need about their disease. Implications for cancer screening and management. Cancer. 1995;**76**(2):167-177

[50] Willis A, Smith S, Meiser B, Ballinger M, Thomas D, Young M. Sociodemographic, psychosocial and clinical factors associated with uptake of genetic counselling for hereditary cancer: A systematic review. Clinical Genetics. 2017;**92**(2):121-133. DOI: 10.1111/cge.12868

[51] Paluch-Shimon S, Cardoso F, Sessa C, Balmana J, Cardoso M, Gilbert F, et al. Prevention and screening in BRCA mutation carriers and other breast/ ovarian hereditary cancer syndromes: ESMO Clinical Practice Guidelines for cancer prevention and screening. Annals of Oncology. 2016;**27**:v103-v110

[52] Bernstein-Molho R, Kaufman B, Ben David M, Sklair-Levy M, Feldman D, Zippel D, et al. Breast cancer for BRCA1/2 mutation carriers – is "early detection" early enough? Breast. 2020;**49**:81-86. DOI: 10.1016/j.breast.2019.10.012

[53] Biglia N, Alonzo M, Sgro L, Cont N, Bounous V, Robba E. Breast cancer treatment in mutation carries: Surgical treatment. Minerva Gynecology. 2016;**68**:548-556

[54] Yamauchi H, Takei J. Management of hereditary breast and ovarian cancer. International Journal of Clinical Oncology. 2017;**23**(1):45-51

[55] Chapgar A. Prophylactic bilateral mastectomy and contralateral prophylactic mastectomy. Surgical Oncology Clinics of North America. 2014;**23**(3):423-430. DOI: 10.1016/j.soc.2014.03.008

[56] Yamauchi H, Nakagawa C, Kobayashi M, Kobayashi Y, Mano T, Nakamura S, et al. Cost-effectiveness of surveillance and prevention strategies in BRCA1/2 mutation carriers. Breast Cancer. 2018;**25**(2):141-150. DOI: 10.1007/s12282-017-0803-y

[57] Schrauder M, Brunel Geuder L, Häberle L, Wunderle M, Hoyer J, Csorba R, et al. Cost effectiveness of bilateral risk-reducing mastectomy and salpingo-oophorectomy. European Journal of Medical Research. 2019;**24**(1):32

[58] Müller D, Danner M, Schmutzeler R, Engel C, Wasserman K, Stollenwerk B, et al. Economic modeling of risk-adapted screen-and-treat strategies in women at high risk for breast or ovarian cancer. The European Journal of Health Economics. 2019;**20**(5):739-750. DOI: 10.1007/s10198-019-01038-1

[59] Heemskerk-Gerritsen B, Brekelmans C, Menke-Pluymers M, van Geel A, Tilanus-Linthorst M, Bartels C, et al. Prophylactic mastectomy in BRCA1/2 mutation carriers and women at risk of hereditary breast cancer: Long-term experiences at the Rotterdam Family Cancer Clinic. Annals of Surgical Oncology.

2007;**14**(12):3335-3344. DOI: 10.1245/s10434-007-9449-x

[60] Rebbeck T, Friebel T, Lynch H, Neuhausen S, et al. Bilateral prophylactic mastectomy reduces breas cancer risk in BRCA1 and BRCA2 mutation carriers: The PROSE Study Group. Journal of Clinical Oncology. 2004;**22**(6):1055-1062. DOI: 10.1200/JCO.2004.04.188

[61] Domchk S, Friebel T, Singer C, Gareth D, Lynch H, Isaacs C, et al. Association of risk-reducing surgery in BRCA1 or BRCA2 mutation carriers with cancer risk and mortality. JAMA. 2010;**304**(9):967-975. DOI: 10.1001/jama.2010.1237

[62] Evans D, Gandhi A, Wisely J, Clancy T, Woodward E, Harvey J, et al. Uptake of bilateral-risk-reducing-mastectomy: Prospective analysis of 7195 women at high-risk of breast cancer. Breast. 2021;**60**:45-52. DOI: 10.1016/j.breast.2021.08.015

[63] Basu NN, Hordon J, Chatterjee S, Gandhi A, Wisely J, Harvey J, et al. The Angelina Jolie effect: Contralateral risk-reducing mastectomy trends in patients at increased risk of breast cancer. Scientific Reports. 2021;**11**(1):2847. DOI: 10.1038/s41598-021-82654-x

[64] Lee J, Kim S, Kang E, Park S, Kim Z, Lee MH, et al. Influence of the Angelina Jolie Announcement and Insurance Reimbursement on Practice Patterns for Hereditary Breast Cancer. J. Breast Cancer. 2017;**20**(2):203-2017

[65] Flippo-Morton T, Walsh K, Chambers K, Amacker-North L, White B, Sarantou T, et al. Surgical decision making in BRCA-positive population: Institutional experience and comparison with recent literature. The Breast Journal. 2016;**22**(1):35-44. DOI: 10.1111/tbj.12521

[66] Rocco N, Montagna G, Criscitiello C, Nava M, Privitera F, Taher W, et al. Nipple sparing mastectomy as a risk-reducing procedure for BRCA-mutated patients. Genes (Basel). 2021;**12**(2):253. DOI: 10.3390/genes12020253

[67] Unukovych D, Sandelin K, Liljegren A, Arver B, Wickman M, Johansson H, et al. Contralateral prophylactic mastectomy in breast cancer patients with a family history: A prospective 2-years follow-up study of health-related quality of life, sexuality and body image. European Cancer. 2012;**48**(17):3150-3156. DOI: 10.1016/j.ejca.2012.04.023

[68] Razdan S, Patel V, Jewell S, McCarthy C. Quality of life among patients after bilateral prophylactic mastectomy: A systematic review of patient-reported outcomes. Quality of Life Research. 2016;**25**(6):1409-1421. DOI: 10.1007/s11136-015-1181-6

[69] Metcalfe K, Esplen MJ, Goel V, Narod S. Psychosocial functioning in women who have undergone bilateral prophylactic mastectomy. Psichooncology. 2004;**13**(1):14-25. DOI: 10.1002/pon.726

[70] Eleje G, Eke A, Ezebialu I, Ikechebeñu J, Ugwu E, Okonkwo O. Risk-reducing bilateral salpingo-oophorectomy in women with BRCA1 or BRCA2 mutations. Cohrane Database System Review. 2018;**8**(8):CD012464. DOI: 10.1002/14651858.CD012464.pub2

[71] Rebbeck T, Kauff N, Domchek S. Meta-analysis of risk reduction estimates associated with risk-reducing salpingo-oophorectomy in BRCA1 or BRCA2 mutation carriers. Journal of the National Cancer Institute. 2009;**102**(2):80-87. DOI: 10.1093/jnci/djn442

[72] Finch A, Metcalfe K, Chiang J, Elit L, Mclaughlin J, Springate C, et al.

The impact of prophylactic salpingo-oophorectomy on quality of life and psychological distress in women with a BRCA mutation. Psichooncology. 2013;**22**(1):212-219. DOI: 10.1002/pon.2401

[73] Gordhandas S, Norquist B, Pennington K, Yung R, Laya M, Swisher E. Hormone replacement therapy after risk reducing salpingo-oophorectomy in patients with BRCA1 or BRCA2 mutations; a systematic review of risks and benefits. Gynecology and Oncology. 2019;**153**(1):192-200

[74] Hickey I, Jha S, Wyld L. The psychosexual effects of risk- reducing bilateral salpingo-oophorectomy in female BRCA1/2 mutation carriers: A systematic review of qualitative studies. Gynecologic Oncology. 2021;**160**(3):763-770. DOI: 10.1016/j.ygyno.2020.12.001

[75] Michelsen T, Dorum A, Tropé C, Fossa S, Dahl A. Fatigue and quality of life after risk-reducing salpingo-oophorectomy in women at increased risk for hereditary breast-ovarian cancer. International Journal of Gynecological Cancer. 2009;**19**(6):1029-1036. DOI: 10.1111/IGC.0b013e3181a83cd5

[76] Finch A, Narod S. Quality of life and health status after prophylactic sapingo-oophorectomy in women who carry a BRCA mutation: A review. Maturitas. 2011;**70**(3):261-265. DOI: 10.1016/j.maturitas.2011.08.001

[77] Glassey R, Ives A, Saunders C, Musiello T. Decision making, psychological wellbeing and psychosocial outcomes for high risk women who choose to undergo bilateral prophylactic mastectomy—A review of the literature. Breast. 2016;**28**:130-135. DOI: 10.1016/j.breast.2016.05.012

[78] Madalinska J, Hollenstein J, Bleiker E, van Beurden M, Valdimarsdottir H, Massuger L, et al. Quality-of-life effects of prophylactic salpingo-oophorectomy versus gynecologic screening among women at increased risk of hereditary ovarian cancer. Journal of Clinical Oncology. 2005;**23**(28):6890-6898. DOI: 10.1200/JCO.2005.02.626

[79] Heemskerk-Gerritsen B, Jager A, Koppert L, Obdeijin A, Collée M, Meijers-Heijboer H, et al. Sarvival after bilateral risk-reducing mastectomy in healthy BRCA1 and BRCA2 mutation carriers. Breast Cancer Research and Treatment. 2019;**177**(3):723-733. DOI: 10.1007/s10549-019-05345-2

[80] Gierej P, Rajca B, Górecki-Gomola A. Bilateral risk- reducing mastectomy—Surgical procedure, complications and financial benefit. Polski Przeglad Chirurgiczny. 2021;**93**(3):1-5. DOI: 10.5604/01.3001.0014.7878

[81] Slade D. PARP and PARG inhibitors in cancer treatment. Genes & Development. 2020;**34**(5-6):360-394. DOI: 10.1101/gad.334516.119

[82] Rosland G, Engelsen A. Novel points of attack for targeted cancer therapy. Basic & Clinical Pharmacology & Toxicology. 2015;**116**(1):9-18. DOI: 10.1111/bcpt.12313

[83] Padma V. An overview of target cancer therapy. Biomedicine (Taipei). 2015;**5**(4):19. DOI: 10.7603/s40681-015-0019-4

[84] Hanahan D, Weinberg R. Hallmarks of cancer: The next generation. Cell. 2011;**144**(5):646-674. DOI: 10.1016/j.cell.2011.02.013

[85] Boussios S, Karihtala P, Moschetta M, Abson C, Karathanasi A, et al. Veliparib in cancer: A new synthetically lethal therapeutic approach. Investigation Drugs. 2020;**38**(1):181-193

[86] Tubbs A, Nussenzweig A. Endogenus DNA damage as a source of genomic instability in cancer. Cell. 2017;**168**(4):644-656. DOI: 10.1016/j.cell.201701.002

[87] Huang R, Zhou P. DNA damage repair: Historical perspectives, mechanistic pathways and clinical translation for target cancer therapy. Signal Transduction and Targeted Therapy. 2021;**6**(1):254. DOI: 10.1038/s41392/s41392-021-00648-7

[88] Fong P, Boss D, Yap T, Tutt A, Wu P, Mergui-Roelvink M, et al. Inhibition of poly(ADP-ribose) polymerase in tumors from BRCA mutation carriers. The New England Journal of Medicine. 2009;**361**(2):123-134. DOI: 10.1056/NEJMoa0900212

[89] Sandhu S, Schelman W, Wilding G, Moreno V, Baird R, Miranda S, et al. The poly(ADP-ribose) polymerase inhibitor niraparib (MK4827) in BRCA mutation carriers and patients with sporadic cancer: A phase 1 dose-escalation trial. Lancet Oncology. 2013;**14**(9):882-892

[90] Kristeleit R, Shapiro G, Burris H, Oza A, LoRusso P, Patel M, et al. A Phase I-II Study the oral PARP inhibitor Rucaparib in patients with Germline BRCA1/2-mutated ovarian carcinoma or other solid tumors. Clinical Cancer Research. 2017;**23**(15):4095-4106

[91] de Bono J et al. Two-Part Trial of the PARP inhibitor talazoparib in patients with advanced germline BRCA1/BRCA2 mutations and selected sporadic cancers. Cancer Discovery. 2017;**7**(6):620-629. DOI: 10.1158/2159-8290.CD-16-1250

[92] Audeh M, Carmichael J, Penson R, Friedlander M, Powell B, Bell-McGuinn M, et al. Oral poly(ADP-ribose) polymerase inhibitor olaparib in patients with BRCA1 or BRCA2 mutations and recurrent ovarian cancer: A proof-of-concept trial. Lancet. 2010;**376**(9737):245-251. DOI: 10.1016/S0140-6736(10)60893-8

[93] Gelmon K, Tischkowitz M, Mackay H, Swenerton K, Robidoux A, Tonkin K, et al. Olaparib in patients with recurrent high-grade serous or poorly differentiated ovarian carcinoma or triple-negative breast cancer: A phase 2, multicentre, open-label, non-randomised study. The Lancet Oncology. 2011;**12**(9):852-861. DOI: 10.1016/S1470-2045(11)70214-5

[94] Kaye S, Matulonis U, Ang J, Gourley C. Phase II, open -label, randomized, multicenter study comparing the efficacy and safety of Olaparib a poly (ADP-ribose) polymerase inhibitor, and pegylated liposomal doxorubicin in patients with BRCA1 or BRCA2 mutations and recurrent ovarian cancer. Journal of Clinical Oncology. 2012;**30**(4):372-379. DOI: 10.1200/JCO.2011.36.9215

[95] Ledermann J, Harter P, Gourley C, Friedlander M, Vergote I, Rustin C, et al. Olaparib maintenance therapy in platinum-sensitive relapsed ovarian cancer. The New England Journal of Medicine. 2012;**366**(15):1382-1392. DOI: 10.1056/NEJMoa1105535

[96] Ledermann J, Harter P, Gourley C, Friedlander M, Vergote I, Rustin C, et al. Olaparib maintenance therapy in patients with platinum-sensitive relapsed serous ovarian cancer: A preplanned retrospective analysis of outcomes by BRCA status in randomised phase 2 trial. The Lancet Oncology. 2014;**15**(8):852-861. DOI: 10.1016/S1470-2045(14)70228-1

[97] Kaufman B, Shapira-Frommer R, Schmutzler R, Audeh M, Friedlancer M, Balmaña J, et al. Olaparib monotherapy in patients with advanced cancer and a

germline BRCA1/2 mutation. Journal of Clinical Oncology. 2015;**33**(3):244-250. DOI: 10.1200/JCO.2014.56.2728

[98] Ledermann J, Harter P, Gourley C, Friedlander M, Vergote I, Rustin C, et al. Overall survival in patients with platinum-sensitive recurrent serous ovarian cancer receiving Olaparib maintenance monotherapy: An update analysis from a randomised, placebo-controlled, double-blind, phase 2 trail. The Lancet Oncology. 2016;**17**(11):1579-1589. DOI: 10.1016/S1470-2045(16)30376-X

[99] Coleman R, Sill M, Bell-McGuinn K, Aghajanian C, Gray H, Tewari K, et al. A phase II evaluation of the potent, highly selective PARP inhibitor veliparib in the treatment of persistent or recurrent epithelial ovarian, fallopian tube, or primary peritoneal cancer in patients who carry a germline BRCA1 or BRCA2 mutation—An NRG Oncology/Gynecologic Oncology Group study. Gynecologic Oncology. 2015;**137**(3):386-391. DOI: 10.1016/j.ygyno.2015.03.042

[100] Robson M, Im S, Senkus E, Xu B, Domchek S, Masuda N, et al. Olaparib for Metastatic Breast cancer in patients with a Germline BRCA Mutation. The New England Journal of Medicine. 2017;**377**(6):523-533. DOI: 10.1056/NEJMoa1706450

[101] Pujade-Lauraine E, Lederman J, Selle F, Gebski V, Person R, et al. Olaparib tablets as maintenance therapy in patients with platinum-sensitive, relapsed ovarian cancer and a BRCA1/mutation (SOLO2/ENGOT-Ov21): A double-blind, ramdomised, placebo controlled, phase 3 trial. The Lancet Oncology. 2017;**18**(9):1274-1284. DOI: 10.1016/S1470-2045(17)30469-2

[102] Moore K, Colombo N, Scambia G, Kim B, Oaknin A, Friedlander M. et al. Maintenance Olaparib in Patients with Newly Diagnosed Advanced Ovarian Cancer. The New England Journal of Medicine. 2018;**379**(26):2495-2505. DOI: 10.1056/NEJMoa1810858

[103] Golan T, Hammel P, Reni M, Van Cutsem E, Macarulla T, Halla M, et al. Maintenance olaparib for germline BRCA-mutated metastatic pancreatic cancer. The New England Journal of Medicine. 2019;**381**(4):317-327. DOI: 10.1056/NEJMoa1903387

[104] Colema R, Oza A, Lorusso D, Aghajanian C, Oaknin A, Dean A, et al. Rucaparib Maintenance treatment for recurrent ovarian carcinoma after response to platinum therapy (ARIEL3): A randomised, double-blind, placebo-controlled, phase 3 trial. Lancet. 2017;**390**(10106):1949-1961

[105] Friedlander M, Gebski V, Gibbs E, Davies L, Bloomfield R, Hilpert F, et al. Health-related quality of life and patient- centred outcomes with Olaparib maintenance after chemotherapy in patients with platinum-sensitive, relapsed ovarian cancer and a BRCA1/2 mutation (SOLO2/ENGOT Ov-21):a placebo—controlled, phase 3 randomised trial. The Lancet Oncology. 2018;**19**(8):1126-1134. DOI: 10.1016/S1470-2045(18)30343-7

[106] Robson M, Ruddy K, Im S, Senkus E, Xi B, Domchek S, et al. Patient-reported outcomes in patients with a germline BRCA mutation and Her2-negative metastatic breast cancer receiving Olaparib versus chemotherapy in the OlympiAD trial. European Journal of Cancer. 2019;**120**:20-30. DOI: 10.1016/j.ejca.2019.06.023